The Cirrhosis Mastery Bible: Your Blueprint for Complete Cirrhosis Management

Dr. Ankita Kashyap and Prof. Krishna N. Sharma

Published by Virtued Press, 2023.

While every precaution has been taken in the preparation of this book, the publisher assumes no responsibility for errors or omissions, or for damages resulting from the use of the information contained herein.

THE CIRRHOSIS MASTERY BIBLE: YOUR BLUEPRINT FOR COMPLETE CIRRHOSIS MANAGEMENT

First edition. December 27, 2023.

ISBN: 979-8223779179

Written by Dr. Ankita Kashyap and Prof. Krishna N. Sharma.

Table of Contents

DISCLAIMER

The information provided in this book is intended for general informational purposes only. The content is not meant to substitute professional medical advice, diagnosis, or treatment. Always consult with a qualified healthcare provider before making any changes to your management plan or healthcare regimen.

While every effort has been made to ensure the accuracy and completeness of the information presented, the author and publisher do not assume any responsibility for errors, omissions, or potential misinterpretations of the content. Individual responses to management strategies may vary, and what works for one person might not be suitable for another.

The book does not endorse any specific medical treatments, products, or services. Readers are encouraged to seek guidance from their healthcare providers to determine the most appropriate approaches for their unique medical conditions and needs.

Any external links or resources provided in the book are for convenience and informational purposes only. The author and publisher do not have control over the content or availability of these external sources and do not endorse or guarantee the accuracy of such information. Readers are advised to exercise caution and use their judgment when applying the information provided in this book to their own situations. The author and publisher disclaim any liability for any direct, indirect, consequential, or other damages arising from the use of this book and its content.

By reading and using this book, readers acknowledge and accept the limitations and inherent risks associated with implementing the strategies, recommendations, and information contained herein. It is always recommended to consult a qualified healthcare professional for personalized medical advice and care.

Introduction

When venturing out onto the terrain of cirrhosis, one may encounter obstacles along the way and a lack of assurance. This, however, is a map—a well designed road map for negotiating the intricacies of this situation with strength and elegance. Welcome to "The Cirrhosis Mastery Bible: Your Blueprint for Complete Cirrhosis Management," where each chapter offers a ray of hope and every phrase serves as a stepping stone toward empowerment.

Picture, if you will, the cells that make up your liver, the hardworking labourers that toil day and night, now overwhelmed by the unrelenting tidal wave of cirrhosis. Yes, it's a war, but you don't have to fight it by yourself. With the help of this guide, you will be armed with a strong information base, a clear grasp of the situation, and useful tactics to help you get your health back.

You might wonder, what is cirrhosis? Let me shed some light on the matter. The end result of persistent liver injury is cirrhosis, which prevents the liver from performing its essential tasks by replacing healthy tissue with scar tissue. Alcohol misuse, hepatitis, and nonalcoholic steatohepatitis are only a few of the numerous reasons, but they all lead to the same problem.

Are you feeling confused by all of the medical terms and the abundance of advise that seems more enigmatic than helpful? Do not be alarmed. This book has straightforward language and concise explanations. Imagine your liver as a filter, a kind of purifier, but one that is now impeded in its capacity to cleanse by scarring. This book breaks down medical jargon and converts it into a conversation that you, the reader, can understand.

You ask, but why this book? There are two parts to the solution: thorough investigation and true empathy. The information contained here is not merely speculation; rather, it is the result of thorough investigation drawn from reputable medical journals and reputable scientific investigations. Every information that is stated is a genuine gem that has been examined and supported by data.

Is it possible for a single book to capture the range of experiences that people with cirrhosis have? Although it may seem like an impossible feat, this volume aims to accomplish just that. Understanding that every trip is different, it provides individualised strategies and self-help methods that fit the specifics of your circumstance.

Allow me to lead you through this page's harmonious fusion of medical and holistic health viewpoints. Imagine a tapestry where each strand is vital to the integrity of the whole and is weaved together with strands of both traditional wisdom and modern medicine.

Maybe you're wondering how to apply these tactics in your day-to-day activities. The solution lies in doable actions and sound guidance with applicability in the actual world. It's about realising how important it is to take care of your health, including what you eat, how you handle stress, and how much sleep you get.

Take a brief break. Think back to what you now know about cirrhosis. Does it seem like a powerful enemy, cloaked in fog? This book is your sunshine, clearing the clouds and bringing the scenery to life in all its detail.

Each chapter you come across has been thoughtfully written so that every page serves as a source of encouragement as well as knowledge. There are narratives that speak to your experience, lists that organise, and diagrams that make sense. The author's tone is one of empathy throughout because she recognises that every instance of cirrhosis is the result of a person with hopes, anxieties, and dreams.

Imagine yourself standing on a beach and looking out over the wide ocean that is cirrhosis management. This book is your ship, built to sail through rough seas and strong winds. I am extremely honoured to have you join us.

Let us get out on this journey together by asking the question that's probably been nagging at the back of your mind the entire time: "Is it possible to live a fulfilling life with cirrhosis?" Turn the page, please, because we are about to embark on a quest to find the solution.

Understanding Cirrhosis

Demystifying Cirrhosis

The first step in understanding cirrhosis is to deconstruct the vocabulary that is necessary to grasp the complexity of this condition. The topography of managing cirrhosis requires a deep comprehension of important terms, each of which acts as a guide across this complex area.

One cannot stress how important it is to comprehend fundamental terms. It is the cornerstone that supports our understanding of cirrhosis. Navigating the huge ocean of cirrhosis management without a thorough understanding of these key words would be like sailing without a compass. Understanding the jargon around cirrhosis provides us with the knowledge necessary to both understand the illness and take proactive measures to treat it.

Before we can begin this trip, we need to recognise and clarify the concepts that serve as the foundation for the management of cirrhosis. The terminology listed below is essential to our comprehension and will act as a road map for our efforts to deconstruct cirrhosis:

1. Cirrhosis: the final stage of long-term liver damage, marked by the scar tissue that replaces healthy liver tissue and lowers liver function.

2. Hepatic Encephalopathy: a reduction in brain function brought on by the liver's incapacity to eliminate toxins from the blood, which causes altered awareness and cognitive impairment.

3. Ascites: the buildup of fluid in the abdomen, which is frequently brought on by liver illness and results in discomfort and swelling there.

4. Portal Hypertension: Elevated intracranial pressure inside the portal vein system, responsible for transporting blood from the intestines to the liver, can result in a number of problems, including hepatic haemorrhage.

5. Hepatocellular Carcinoma: a kind of liver cancer that poses serious management and treatment challenges since it frequently develops in the context of cirrhosis.

Cirrhosis: The gradual and irreversible liver disease cirrhosis is typified by the formation of scar tissue in lieu of healthy liver tissue. The liver's regular structure is upset by this scarring, which makes it more difficult for the organ to perform vital processes including metabolism, detoxification, and the synthesis of proteins required for blood clotting.

Hepatic Encephalopathy: The accumulation of ammonia in the bloodstream due to the liver's incapacity to eliminate toxins from the bloodstream causes hepatic encephalopathy, a consequence of advanced liver disease that impairs brain function. Numerous neurological symptoms, such as disorientation, confusion, and in extreme situations, coma, may result from this.

Ascites: The buildup of fluid in the abdominal cavity, known as ascites, is frequently brought on by cirrhosis. The body's fluid balance is upset by the compromised liver function, which results in an accumulation of fluid in the abdomen and breathing difficulties.

Portal Hypertension: Increased pressure in the portal venous system, which transports blood from the digestive organs to the liver, is a defining feature of portal hypertension. Varices, which are dilated blood veins in the stomach or oesophagus that are prone to bleeding, can develop as a result of this increased pressure and pose a serious risk to people with cirrhosis.

Hepatocellular Carcinoma: The most prevalent kind of primary liver cancer, hepatocellular carcinoma, frequently develops in the context of cirrhosis. Because cirrhosis raises the risk of hepatocellular carcinoma, early identification and routine observation are essential for successful treatment.

It can be intimidating to understand these technical medical jargon, but making comparisons to more familiar ideas can help with understanding. Think of the liver as a busy factory, where the cells are hard at work keeping the body's internal equilibrium. When cirrhosis is present, the factory gets burdened by scar tissue, which prevents it from operating at peak efficiency. This comparison offers a realistic framework for comprehending how cirrhosis affects the essential processes of the liver.

Ascites can be compared to a soggy garden, where the surplus fluid in the abdomen represents the uneven distribution of water in the soil. This analogy provides a concrete illustration of cirrhosis by drawing a parallel between the buildup of fluid in the belly and the difficulties experienced by those who have the illness.

Moreover, portal hypertension can be thought of as a bottleneck in the blood arteries of the liver, similar to a jammed highway that results in elevated pressure in the portal vein system. This analogy helps to clarify the intricacies of cirrhosis by offering a practical connection to the physiological alterations taking place in the liver.

Conclusion:

Understanding the basic language that guides this path is essential as we explore the field of cirrhosis management. Through deciphering the essential terminology linked to cirrhosis, we facilitate a more profound understanding of the illness and enable ourselves to effectively and intelligently navigate the intricacies of managing cirrhosis.

Signs and Signals

When it comes to managing cirrhosis, it is critical to identify the early warning signs and symptoms that are vital markers of the changing disease. By being able to recognise these cues, people and medical professionals can take proactive measures to slow the advancement of cirrhosis and improve patient care. By outlining the crucial symptoms and indicators of cirrhosis, this extensive list seeks to provide a path for early detection and treatment.

The cardinal indications and signals of cirrhosis are listed below, highlighting the condition's complexity and emphasising the need for awareness while identifying various manifestations:

1. Jaundice: a characteristic yellowing of the eyes and skin that denotes hepatic impairment.

2. Fatigue and Weakness: weariness and decreased endurance, which are indicative of the systemic effects of cirrhosis on the body.

3. Abdominal Swelling: the buildup of fluid in the abdominal cavity, which causes discomfort and distension.

4. Easy Bruising and Bleeding: heightened bruising and bleeding susceptibility, suggesting impaired blood clotting function.

5. Mental Confusion: Hepatic encephalopathy resulting in reduced mental sharpness and cognitive impairment.

6. Spider Angiomas: spider-like blood veins that are visible on the skin and are indicative of liver disease.

7. Unexplained Weight Loss: unintended weight reduction that indicates metabolic problems even in the face of a stable food and way of life.

8. Itchy Skin: chronic itching brought on by an accumulation of toxins in the blood, which is indicative of liver damage.

a. The buildup of the yellow pigment bilirubin in the body causes jaundice, which is marked by the yellowing of the skin and eyes. When bilirubin is not metabolised and excreted properly in the context of cirrhosis, it builds up in the blood and eventually shows up in the sclera and skin. This visual cue is a clear sign of liver disease and should be evaluated by medical specialists as soon as possible.

b. The systemic effects of liver damage are the cause of the widespread weakness and exhaustion that cirrhosis patients suffer. The liver is essential for the metabolism of energy and the storage of nutrients; cirrhosis impairs the liver's ability to do these functions, making it less able to maintain adequate energy levels. Moreover, the effects of cirrhosis on the body's general metabolic equilibrium add to the extreme exhaustion and weakness that afflicted people endure.

c. One of the main signs of advanced cirrhosis is ascites, or the buildup of fluid in the abdominal cavity. The hepatic portal vein system's high pressure combined with the liver's decreased ability to synthesise proteins causes the peritoneal cavity to fill with fluid. For individuals afflicted, this distension in the abdomen not only signals the advancement of cirrhosis but also causes great agony and limits their ability to work.

d. Prolonged bleeding and easy bruising are made more likely by the liver's impaired ability to synthesise clotting components in cirrhosis. Increased susceptibility to bruising and bleeding is caused by a combination of factors including platelet dysfunction, reduced clotting factor production, and altered vascular dynamics. As such, it is important to monitor and manage these hemostatic issues carefully.

e. The result of severe liver illness, hepatic encephalopathy causes cognitive decline, altered consciousness, and behavioural abnormalities. The build-up of neurotoxins, especially ammonia, in the blood causes the brain to be affected neurotoxically, which causes the typical mental disorientation and neuropsychiatric symptoms that people with cirrhosis experience. In order to lessen the negative effects of hepatic encephalopathy on patient outcomes, early detection and treatment are essential.

f. Spider angiomas, sometimes known as spider nevi, are a dermatological sign indicating underlying liver disease. These unique vascular lesions, which have a central arteriole encircled by smaller capillaries, are indicative of the altered vascular dynamics and vasodilatory disruptions that are intrinsic to cirrhosis.

g. Inadvertent weight loss in the context of cirrhosis is a reflection of affected people's decreased dietary status and metabolic dysregulation. A thorough evaluation of nutritional status and metabolic needs is necessary since advanced cirrhosis patients experience unexplained weight loss that is attributed to a combination of reduced caloric intake, impaired nutrient absorption, and metabolic inefficiencies.

h. One of the most prevalent and upsetting symptoms of cirrhosis is pruritus, or continuous itching, which is caused by the buildup of bile salts and other toxins in the blood. These pruritogenic chemicals are retained by the liver due to reduced excretory activity, resulting in the typical itching that severely reduces the quality of life for cirrhosis patients.

The importance of these indicators and signals in the context of cirrhosis is supported by research investigations and clinical observations. Several studies have demonstrated the diagnostic and prognostic significance of hepatic encephalopathy, ascites, and jaundice in predicting patient outcomes and the severity of the disease. Moreover, first-person testimonies from cirrhosis patients highlight the significant influence these symptoms have on their day-to-day activities and stress the need of early detection and treatment.

The clinical evaluation and treatment of cirrhosis depend heavily on the identification and comprehension of these indicators. In order to enable prompt intervention and individualised care, healthcare providers need to be alert in eliciting and assessing these manifestations during patient contacts. Furthermore, those who have been diagnosed with or at risk for cirrhosis gain from having a greater awareness of these early warning indicators since it enables them to take proactive self-care practises and seek prompt medical intervention.

As we move from the explanation of these essential symptoms and indicators to the next section that deals with diagnostic techniques and treatments, it is critical to acknowledge the connection between these components in the overall care of cirrhosis. The key to improving patient outcomes and raising the standard of cirrhosis care is the smooth integration of early detection, precise diagnosis, and focused therapy.

This in-depth examination of the early warning indicators and symptoms of cirrhosis not only clarifies the complex nature of this illness but also emphasises the necessity of being watchful and proactive in managing it. The ability to identify and understand these vital indicators and signals is crucial for navigating the intricacies of cirrhosis. It illuminates the route toward early detection, intervention, and the improvement of patient well-being.

Unraveling the Causes

Chronic and progressive liver disease cirrhosis is a major global health concern that affects afflicted individuals as well as healthcare systems globally. Due to the complex interaction between etiological variables and pathophysiological mechanisms, cirrhosis is a multifactorial disease that necessitates a thorough knowledge of its various risk factors and causes. In order to provide insight into the complex landscape of cirrhosis and to emphasise the need of early detection and targeted preventive measures, this chapter attempts to disentangle the intricate network of causative agents and predisposing factors that lead to the development and progression of the condition.

Cirrhosis originates from a variety of etiological events that lead to persistent liver injury, which in turn causes gradual distortion of the hepatic architecture, compromise of function, and the appearance of clinical consequences. The confluence of several etiologies, including metabolic disorders, viral infections, long-term alcohol use, and autoimmune mechanisms, among others, highlights the complexity and heterogeneity of the cirrhosis causal landscape. Therefore, a detailed explanation of these contributing factors is essential to promoting a comprehensive management strategy for cirrhosis that includes preventive measures, customised interventions, and focused surveillance tactics.

The complex interactions among the components that cause cirrhosis result in a range of significant outcomes, including the gradual development of liver fibrosis, as well as the onset of decompensated liver disease, portal hypertension, and hepatocellular cancer. The unrelenting progression of cirrhosis sustains a series of systemic symptoms, including hepatic encephalopathy, ascites, variceal haemorrhage, and hepatorenal syndrome, all of which have an impact on the life expectancy, functional ability, and general survival of those who are impacted. Furthermore, the socioeconomic cost of cirrhosis highlights the condition's far-reaching effects on people, families, and healthcare systems. This cost includes healthcare use, lost productivity at work, and the necessity of liver transplantation.

Preventive techniques, early interventions, and tailored surveillance measures are critical in addressing the intricate web of cirrhosis etiologies and risk factors. Comprehensive public health efforts, including alcohol harm reduction programmes, metabolic syndrome management, and viral hepatitis immunisation campaigns, are essential steps in reducing the prevalence of cirrhosis in the general population. Personalized approach to cirrhosis prevention and management is further supported by the targeted identification and tailored management of particular etiological variables, such as immunomodulatory drugs, lifestyle adjustments, and antiviral medications.

Adopting preventive techniques and focused interventions requires a multifaceted strategy that includes public health campaigns, training for healthcare providers, and customised patient care. The cornerstone of preventive care is the smooth integration of hepatitis B and C vaccination programmes, increased knowledge of alcohol-related liver disease, and early identification of metabolic risk factors in clinical encounters. Moreover, a customised and interdisciplinary approach to patient care is necessary for the personalised application of etiology-specific interventions, such as antiviral treatments, immunosuppressive regimens, and nutritional assistance.

When preventative measures and focused interventions are used wisely, the results in cirrhosis can be extensive and include reduction of disease burden, reduction of liver-related morbidity and death, and enhancement of patient quality of life. Clinical observations and epidemiological data highlight the importance of early metabolic syndrome management in preventing the development of non-alcoholic fatty liver disease-related cirrhosis, the effectiveness of alcohol harm reduction programmes in slowing the progression of alcoholic liver disease, and the effectiveness of vaccination campaigns in lowering the incidence of viral hepatitis-related cirrhosis. Moreover, the tailored application of etiology-specific interventions, such as immunosuppressive regimens, antiviral therapies, and nutritional support, results in positive outcomes concerning the stabilisation of the disease, improvement of function, and reduction of complications related to the liver.

Other approaches to treating cirrhosis etiologies and risk factors include a careful investigation of new therapeutic modalities such as immunomodulatory drugs, focused pharmacotherapies, and precision medicine techniques. The expanding field of study in microbiome regulation, disease-specific molecular targets, and precision nutrition signals a potentially fruitful path toward the customised treatment of cirrhosis etiologies, which emphasises the necessity of continued investigation and translational efforts in this area. In addition, the incorporation of comprehensive lifestyle adjustments, which include dietary treatments, exercise routines, and stress reduction techniques, represents an additional pathway for the avoidance and treatment of cirrhosis associated with metabolic syndrome, highlighting the complex character of prophylactic actions in this regard.

As we move from the detailed dissection of cirrhosis etiologies and risk factors to the following sections discussing therapeutic interventions, diagnostic modalities, and ongoing research projects, it is critical to acknowledge the interdependence of these components in the overall management of cirrhosis. Optimizing patient outcomes, reducing disease burden, and improving the standard of cirrhosis therapy are all dependent on the smooth integration of etiology-specific prevention initiatives, precise diagnostic methods, and focused interventions.

In addition to shedding light on the complex nature of cirrhosis, this thorough investigation of its origins and risk factors emphasises the significance of early detection, focused surveillance, and preventative approaches in reducing the illness burden and enhancing patient outcomes. Clarifying these risk variables and causal factors helps us traverse the intricacies of cirrhosis by providing a compass that points the way toward preventive awareness, tailored therapies, and the best possible care of the disease.

Stages of Severity

To provide the reader with a thorough picture of the disease's progressive nature, it is important to comprehend the many levels of severity associated with cirrhosis. The reader will obtain an understanding of the changing clinical symptoms, prognostic implications, and the necessity of specific interventions at each stage by outlining the many phases of cirrhosis and its consequences.

Readers need have a basic awareness of liver anatomy, hepatic function, and the pathophysiological basis of cirrhosis in order to understand the stages of severity in the disease. Understanding the clinical terms and diagnostic techniques used in the evaluation of cirrhosis will also improve understanding of the information provided.

There are multiple discrete stages in which cirrhosis progresses, each with unique histological alterations, clinical presentations, and prognostic consequences. The progressive development of compensated to decompensated cirrhosis signals a change in the state from subclinical illness to overt hepatic decompensation, which results in a variety of systemic symptoms and an increased mortality risk.

The progression of cirrhosis is characterised by multiple phases, the first of which is the compensated phase, during which the liver function is preserved and fibrotic nodules gradually grow. A more severe phase of the disease is marked by the emergence of clinical problems such as ascites, hepatic encephalopathy, variceal bleeding, and hepatorenal syndrome, which are heralded by the start of decompensated cirrhosis as the disease progresses. The following stages include the development of end-stage liver disease, portal vein thrombosis, and hepatocellular carcinoma, each with unique clinical and prognosis implications.

Regular surveillance is essential for people with cirrhosis in order to discover problems early on, such as hepatocellular cancer, esophageal varices, and hepatic encephalopathy. Prompt measures, including medication therapy, endoscopic procedures, and examination of liver transplantation, are essential for slowing the progression of cirrhosis and improving the prognosis of patients. Furthermore, maintaining liver function and preventing the course of disease require abstaining from hepatotoxic drugs such as alcohol and some pharmaceuticals.

An extensive assessment of portal hypertension, hepatic synthetic function, and the existence of clinical consequences are required to determine the severity of cirrhosis. The foundation of illness staging and prognosis include diagnostic modalities such as liver function tests, imaging investigations, endoscopic examinations, and non-invasive fibrosis assessments. Prognostic ratings, such as the Model for End-Stage Liver Disease (MELD) and Child-Turcotte-Pugh scores, also help guide treatment decisions by providing important information about the severity of the disease.

The precise evaluation of disease stage, the prediction of clinical consequences, and the prompt identification of disease progression can all present common issues in the context of the severity of cirrhosis. The management of cirrhosis can be optimised throughout its evolving stages by close coordination with hepatology specialists, prudent use of sophisticated imaging modalities, and integration of multidisciplinary care teams. These strategies can help to reduce these issues.

As we break down the severity stages of cirrhosis, it becomes clear that because the disease is progressing, it is important to have a sophisticated grasp of how the clinical landscape is changing and to implement customised therapies at each step. Through an exploration of the various phases and their consequences, readers will acquire a thorough understanding of the progression of cirrhosis, which will support the necessity of close monitoring, prompt treatment, and the enhancement of patient outcomes.

The Diagnosis Journey

Giving the reader a thorough grasp of the medical tests and methods used in cirrhosis diagnosis is the aim of the diagnosis journey. The reader will obtain an understanding of the critical significance that a fast and correct diagnosis plays in enabling appropriate management and therapy interventions for cirrhosis by reading this description of the sequential processes involved in the diagnostic process.

Readers should have a basic awareness of liver architecture, the pathophysiological basis of cirrhosis, and familiarity with clinical terminology and diagnostic modalities utilised in the assessment of liver disease in order to fully comprehend the diagnosis journey in cirrhosis. Furthermore, a rudimentary awareness of the laboratory tests, imaging investigations, and invasive procedures that are frequently used to diagnose cirrhosis will improve understanding of the information that is presented.

The path to a diagnosis of cirrhosis involves a wide range of diagnostic tests and procedures designed to identify the cause of liver disease, confirm the existence of cirrhosis, assess for complications, and inform treatment decisions. This technique entails a methodical, step-by-step approach that starts with non-invasive testing and advances to more invasive modalities when needed. The end goal is to formulate an accurate diagnosis and initiate focused therapy.

A complete clinical assessment that includes a detailed medical history, physical examination, and risk factor evaluation for liver disease is the first step in the diagnosis process for cirrhosis. After that, non-invasive diagnostic procedures such as liver function tests, serological markers, and imaging studies like CT, MRI, and ultrasound are used to determine the liver's structure, check for cirrhosis and fibrosis, and identify complications like portal hypertension and hepatocellular carcinoma. When non-invasive testing are unable to provide a clear diagnosis or when accurate liver histology is required, invasive techniques like liver biopsy or transient elastography may be necessary to confirm the diagnosis and direct treatment plans. Furthermore, a crucial component of the diagnostic procedure is the evaluation for cirrhosis consequences, such as esophageal varices, ascites, hepatic encephalopathy, and hepatorenal syndrome, which inform cirrhosis management and prognosis.

In order to diagnose cirrhosis, medical professionals must use a methodical and complete approach that includes a thorough clinical examination, the prudent use of non-invasive testing, and the prompt use of invasive procedures where necessary. The examination of consequences warrants close attention since prompt identification of decompensated cirrhosis and related clinical manifestations is essential for informing treatment decisions and enhancing patient outcomes. Furthermore, to ensure the precise diagnosis and customised management of cirrhosis, careful interpretation of diagnostic results, close coordination with hepatology specialists, and integration of multidisciplinary care teams are necessary.

A thorough examination of all diagnostic data, such as liver function tests, imaging studies, histology results from liver biopsies, and transient elastography, is necessary to validate the diagnosis of cirrhosis. The foundation of disease validation and the process of formulating an accurate diagnosis are formed by the correlation of these results with the clinical presentation and the evaluation for complications of cirrhosis. In addition, the application of prognostic metrics, such as the MELD score, facilitates risk assessment and therapy choice, guiding the necessity of liver transplant assessment and improving patient outcomes.

Common difficulties in the context of the cirrhosis diagnosis process can include accurately interpreting test results, assessing for complications, and promptly identifying the cause of the disease. The implementation of multidisciplinary care teams, careful use of advanced imaging modalities, and close coordination with hepatology specialists can all help to minimise these difficulties and streamline the diagnostic process, ultimately leading to the development of a precise diagnosis and the start of focused interventions.

As we begin the process of diagnosing cirrhosis, it is clear that careful assessment of diagnostic tests and procedures is essential to determining whether cirrhosis is present, directing treatment, and improving patient outcomes. Through outlining the successive steps that make up the diagnosis journey, readers will acquire a thorough understanding of the critical role that a timely and accurate diagnosis plays in managing cirrhosis, which in turn supports the necessity of individualised interventions and the enhancement of patient care.

Common Misconceptions

As one of the main causes of chronic liver disease and liver-related death, cirrhosis affects about 4.5 million people in the United States alone. This concerning figure highlights the extensive effects of cirrhosis and the pressing requirement for all-encompassing management approaches to deal with this serious health issue.

In addition to its startlingly high incidence, cirrhosis has a significant impact on people's lives and the lives of their families. It can present with a variety of clinical presentations, from mild symptoms to potentially fatal consequences. Healthcare professionals as well as those who are at risk of liver disease or have been diagnosed with cirrhosis must comprehend the extensive consequences of the condition.

The more we learn about the complexity of cirrhosis, the more obvious it is that medical interventions are not the only way that disease is managed. It emphasises the necessity for a thorough and individualised approach to cirrhosis care and covers lifestyle changes, nutritional concerns, psychological support, and holistic approaches to wellbeing. The severe effects of cirrhosis on a person's physical, mental, and social well-being emphasise the need for multimodal therapies that take into account the various facets of the illness.

The startlingly high incidence of cirrhosis raises important concerns regarding the underlying causes of its increase and possible preventative measures. What are the underlying causes of cirrhosis, and what steps can people take to lower their chance of contracting this crippling illness? Moreover, what all-encompassing strategies may be implemented to empower cirrhosis patients and improve their quality of life?

The educational trip provided by "The Cirrhosis Mastery Bible: Your Blueprint for Complete Cirrhosis Management" is bridged by the revelations of cirrhosis. This book takes readers on a thorough exploration of the many facets of cirrhosis and offers a comprehensive care plan that takes into account lifestyle, diet, medicine, and psychology. It does this by dispelling myths and realities surrounding cirrhosis.

Dr. Ankita Kashyap, a physician and health and wellness coach, is the author of "The Cirrhosis Mastery Bible: Your Blueprint for Complete Cirrhosis Management." She is dedicated to demystifying the complexities of cirrhosis and equipping people with the information and resources they need to overcome the obstacles this condition presents. Dr. Kashyap promotes a holistic approach to healthcare with her team of specialists from various health and wellness fields. She emphasises the integration of dietary planning, psychological techniques, self-care strategies, counselling, lifestyle modifications, and coping mechanisms in the management of cirrhosis.

The frequency of cirrhosis and its effects on people as well as communities highlight how important it is to debunk myths and promote a better knowledge of this illness. With the help of this book, readers will set out on a life-changing path that goes beyond simply managing cirrhosis and includes developing holistic well-being in the midst of this difficult illness.

We shall examine the complexities of cirrhosis in the upcoming chapters, starting with an examination of its pathophysiological foundations, associated risk factors, and clinical presentations. Readers will learn about the many facets of cirrhosis and its various manifestations by dissecting the intricate interaction of elements that contribute to the disease.

Next, we shall traverse the terrain of managing cirrhosis, which includes medical therapies, dietary concerns, psychological assistance, and lifestyle adjustments. Readers will receive thorough counsel that is customised to meet their specific needs, giving them the knowledge and tools they need to address the various aspects of cirrhosis and improve their quality of life.

This book will also shed light on the critical role that multidisciplinary care plays in the management of cirrhosis, as well as the cooperative efforts of medical experts. Readers will obtain a thorough understanding of the holistic approach needed to address the complicated requirements of people living with cirrhosis by cultivating an appreciation of the interconnectivity of multiple healthcare areas.

With a thorough grasp of cirrhosis, readers of "The Cirrhosis Mastery Bible: Your Blueprint for Complete Cirrhosis Management" will be equipped to dispel common myths and take a revolutionary step toward holistic well-being. Leading this journey are Dr. Ankita Kashyap and her team of professionals, who are dedicated to assisting and mentoring people in their quest for the best possible health and well-being while having cirrhosis.

This book is more than just a collection of medical knowledge; it's a source of inspiration, an empowerment manual, and evidence of the possibility and resiliency of holistic healing even in the face of difficult medical circumstances. Come along with us as we set out on this life-changing adventure to understand the complexity of cirrhosis and open the door to complete cirrhosis management and overall wellbeing.

Cirrhosis and Co-morbidities

Chronic liver disease called cirrhosis, which is defined by the replacement of good liver tissue with scar tissue, has a major effect on an individual's general health and frequently results in a multitude of co-morbidities that add a great deal to the complexity of managing this illness. The way that cirrhosis and its co-morbidities interact highlights the importance of having a thorough grasp of these complex interactions and their wider ramifications. This chapter will explore the complex network of co-morbidities linked to cirrhosis, highlighting the parallels and discrepancies between them and providing an understanding of the various facets of managing cirrhosis.

Numerous co-morbidities, such as portal hypertension, ascites, hepatic encephalopathy, hepatorenal syndrome, and hepatocellular cancer, are frequently linked to cirrhosis. The management of cirrhosis is complicated by each of these co-morbidities, which has a substantial effect on the prognosis and quality of life of those who have it. Healthcare professionals and those who have cirrhosis must comprehend the intricate interactions that exist between the disease and its co-morbidities.

The purpose of comparing cirrhosis and its co-morbidities is to clarify how these illnesses are related to one another and how they together affect people's health and quality of life. This analysis aims to offer insights into the holistic care of cirrhosis and its related co-morbidities by comparing and contrasting them. This will promote a comprehensive strategy that takes into account the various aspects of this complicated disease.

The pathophysiological processes, clinical manifestations, therapeutic approaches, and prognostic consequences of cirrhosis and associated co-morbidities will all be included in the comparative standards. We can clarify the complex relationships and illuminate the wider ramifications of their interactions by defining these parameters.

Portal hypertension and cirrhosis are closely related conditions because cirrhosis in particular is frequently accompanied by portal hypertension. Varices, ascites, and other problems can arise as a result of portal hypertension, which is brought on by the increased resistance to portal blood flow in cirrhosis. As an example of how these illnesses are interlinked, ascites, a typical consequence of cirrhosis, can also be linked to the underlying portal hypertension.

Another serious co-morbidity of cirrhosis is hepatic encephalopathy, which is characterised by impaired brain function from the build-up of toxins in the bloodstream that the liver is normally responsible for filtering. The emergence of hepatic encephalopathy in patients with cirrhosis highlights the complex interplay between liver function and neurological symptoms, calling for a multidisciplinary approach to the disease's management that takes into account both the neurological consequences and the underlying liver disease.

Further highlighting the systemic effects of cirrhosis and the complex relationships between liver and renal physiology is hepatorenal syndrome, a major consequence of cirrhosis defined by the progressive degradation of kidney function. Comprehensive therapies that target the hepatic and renal elements of this co-morbidity are necessary, as the therapy of hepatorenal syndrome presents distinct obstacles.

Moreover, the elevated likelihood of hepatocellular carcinoma in cirrhotic persons underscores the significant consequences of this co-morbidity on the general prognosis and enduring results of cirrhotic patients. The complex interrelationship between hepatocellular carcinoma and cirrhosis highlights the need for early detection, surveillance, and comprehensive care approaches to lessen the consequences of this potentially lethal condition.

Although cirrhosis and its co-morbidities have similar pathophysiological causes, they differ in their clinical presentation, treatment options, and prognostic significance, requiring customised approaches to each condition's management. For example, although portal hypertension and cirrhosis are closely related conditions, the treatment of portal hypertension specifically may entail different approaches, such as the use of beta-blockers, endoscopic variceal ligation, transjugular intrahepatic portosystemic shunt (TIPS), or surgical shunts, from the more general management of cirrhosis.

Similar to this, the treatment of ascites in cirrhosis includes diuretic therapy, dietary sodium restriction, and in cases of refractory treatment, paracentesis or transjugular intrahepatic portosystemic shunt (TIPS). This highlights the complex strategy needed to address this particular co-morbidity within the larger framework of managing cirrhosis.

Hepatic encephalopathy requires treatments aimed at lowering ammonia levels, such as rifaximin and lactulose, in addition to liver function optimization; this underscores the unique factors to be taken into account when managing this neurological complication within the context of cirrhosis therapy.

Different from the general management of cirrhosis, the management of hepatorenal syndrome may involve specific vasoconstrictor and albumin infusion therapies to improve renal perfusion. This highlights the need for targeted interventions that address the distinct pathophysiological mechanisms underlying this co-morbidity.

Additionally, the management of this co-morbidity differs from the more general approaches used for cirrhosis itself due to the need for specialised approaches that include imaging studies, tumour staging, and multidisciplinary interventions for the surveillance, early detection, and treatment modalities for hepatocellular carcinoma in cirrhotic patients.

To clearly and concisely illustrate the connections and distinctions between cirrhosis and its co-morbidities, visual aids like flowcharts, diagrams, and comparative tables can be used to highlight the parallels and differences between the two conditions.

The contrasts and parallels between cirrhosis and its co-morbidities highlight the complex network of relationships and the multidimensional approach to treating this complicated illness. The pathophysiological pathways that are interrelated highlight the systemic impact of cirrhosis, making a thorough understanding of its co-morbidities and their implications for holistic management imperative.

The complex interrelationships between co-morbidities and cirrhosis highlight the need for multidisciplinary care that addresses the various aspects of this condition. This care should involve hepatology, gastroenterology, nephrology, neurology, oncology, and other specialised fields to provide comprehensive and individualised interventions that are suited to each patient's unique needs.

Additionally, the various clinical presentations and management techniques associated with cirrhosis and its co-morbidities highlight the necessity of customised strategies that acknowledge the particular difficulties presented by each complication, highlighting the significance of personalised care plans that cater to the particular requirements of those who are impacted.

The contrasts and similarities between cirrhosis and its co-morbidities are highly relevant now given the field's advancements in medicine, technology, and treatment approaches. The comparisons provide valuable insights that support ongoing efforts to improve treatment algorithms, clinical practise standards, and the quality of care for patients with cirrhosis and related co-morbidities.

To sum up, the examination of cirrhosis and its associated disorders provides important understanding of how these illnesses are related to one another and how they affect the overall health and quality of life of those who are impacted. Healthcare professionals and patients can develop a thorough understanding of the complex aspects of managing cirrhosis by identifying the similarities and differences between them and exploring the wider implications of their interactions. This will open the door to comprehensive care that takes into account the various complexities of the condition.

Medical Treatments Unveiled

Medication Management

The characteristic of cirrhosis, a chronic and progressive liver disease, is the replacement of healthy liver tissue with scar tissue. The liver's capacity to operate normally is hampered by growing scarring, which can result in a number of issues. A complete approach is necessary for the care of cirrhosis, with medication being a key component in managing symptoms, preventing complications, and enhancing overall quality of life. We will examine the complexities of medication management in cirrhosis in this chapter, including the many pharmaceutical interventions, how they work, and how they affect the course of the illness.

Medication is used in cirrhosis therapy in a variety of ways to treat a broad range of symptoms and problems resulting from liver failure. Reducing symptoms that negatively affect a person with cirrhosis's quality of life, like weariness, itching, and stomach discomfort, is one of the main objectives of drug treatment. Furthermore, pharmaceuticals are used to treat problems such ascites, hepatic encephalopathy, and variceal haemorrhage, which can be fatal if untreated.

Moreover, pharmaceutical therapies are essential for addressing the fundamental mechanisms behind the advancement of cirrhosis. For example, several drugs target fibrosis and inflammation in an effort to decrease the risk of decompensation and halt the course of liver scarring. Comprehending the mechanisms of action of these drugs is crucial to understanding their function in managing cirrhosis and their possible influence on the course of the illness.

Consider the scenario of a patient presenting with ascites, a frequent consequence of advanced liver disease, to demonstrate the practical use of drug management in cirrhosis. Diuretics, such furosemide and spironolactone, are frequently administered to treat ascites and lessen fluid retention. Optimizing the therapeutic success for these patients mostly depends on knowing the right dosage, keeping an eye out for any adverse effects, and identifying the symptoms of diuretic resistance.

The treatment of hepatic encephalopathy, a neuropsychiatric side effect of cirrhosis, is another example. Non-absorbable disaccharide cellulose is frequently used to encourage the excretion of ammonia, which is a major factor in the development of encephalopathy. Patients and caregivers can understand the logic for lactulose's inclusion in the treatment regimen better if it is explained how it lowers ammonia levels and enhances cognitive function.

When thinking about drug management in cirrhosis, it is important to recognise the various viewpoints that are present in this intricate field. As far as healthcare practitioners are concerned, the focus is on individualised medicine plans that take into account the needs of each patient, taking into account things like liver function, comorbidities, and possible drug interactions. Incorporating patient perspectives is equally important because people with cirrhosis may have different experiences with medications. These experiences might range from worries about side effects to the expense of prescription drugs.

Furthermore, the importance of family members and caregivers in medicine administration cannot be overstated. Optimizing treatment adherence and reducing the risk of adverse events requires educating and incorporating these stakeholders in the administration and monitoring of drugs. Through the presentation of these many viewpoints, a more comprehensive knowledge of the administration of medication in cirrhosis is revealed, emphasising the interdependence of healthcare stakeholders in the pursuit of the best possible patient outcomes.

Facts and evidence-based data are crucial in supporting the safety and effectiveness of drugs used in the treatment of cirrhosis. For example, beta-blockers are effective in lowering the incidence of variceal bleeding in cirrhotic individuals with high-risk esophageal varices, according to a systematic analysis of randomised controlled trials. Citing particular research and their results strengthens the case for using beta-blockers as a preventative measure and establishes their empirical basis.

In a similar vein, facts about medication adherence and how it affects the course of disease can be included to emphasise how crucial it is to follow recommended regimens. A quantitative viewpoint on the significant influence of pharmacological therapies in the management of cirrhosis can be obtained by highlighting data related to the decrease in hospitalizations and increases in overall survival linked with medication adherence.

A number of technical phrases and jargon related to drug management may be difficult for patients and caregivers to understand. For example, the notion of pharmacokinetics, which includes medication distribution, metabolism, excretion, and absorption, might be especially intimidating to those who are not familiar with these concepts. The complexities of medicine dosing and monitoring are made more understandable and accessible to a wider audience by demystifying these ideas.

Additionally, by making terminology linked to possible drug interactions and side effects more understandable, patients and caregivers will be better able to identify and report worrying symptoms, improving the safety and effectiveness of treatment. People facing cirrhosis management can make educated decisions and actively engage in their treatment path by being given clear grasp of medication-related ideas and by having difficult phrases demystified.

In summary, medication management plays a complex and crucial role in controlling complications, treating symptoms, and influencing the course of the illness in cirrhosis. A deeper comprehension of drug management in cirrhosis is revealed by thoroughly outlining the principles, offering real-world examples, investigating various viewpoints, incorporating data and facts, deciphering technical words, and highlighting important takeaways. In the end, this information gives people the understanding and confidence to handle the intricacies of drug schedules, leading to the best possible outcomes in the treatment of cirrhosis.

Navigating Liver Transplantation

For patients with severe cirrhosis, liver transplantation is an essential therapeutic option that may extend survival time and enhance quality of life. Liver transplantation is a complicated process that includes careful evaluation methods, strict patient selection criteria, and extensive post-transplant care. We will explore the complexities of liver transplantation in this chapter, offering details on the procedure, requirements, and recuperation in the process of giving readers a thorough grasp of this life-changing medical procedure.

The surgical replacement of a sick liver with a healthy liver from a deceased or living donor is referred to as liver transplantation. This technique offers patients with severe cirrhosis the opportunity to regain liver function and resume their life without the limitations imposed by their failing liver health. It is a final treatment for end-stage liver disease. Liver transplantation is a complete procedure that goes beyond surgery to include pre-transplant evaluation, donor matching, surgical transplantation, and long-term after-transplant care.

Comprehending the intricacies of this intervention requires an in-depth investigation of the transplant candidate selection criteria, the organ allocation process, the actual surgical surgery, and the continued monitoring of the recipient's health after transplantation. By clarifying the various aspects of liver transplantation, those who are going through this process can better understand the scope of this life-changing procedure and the factors that are essential to its success.

Examine the scenario of a patient who fits the requirements for liver transplantation and has decompensated cirrhosis to demonstrate the practical application of navigating liver transplantation. The first stage entails a thorough assessment to determine whether the patient is a good candidate for transplantation. This evaluation includes a psychosocial assessment, a liver function assessment, and a comorbidity assessment. These evaluations are essential in establishing the patient's eligibility for transplantation and maximising their results following the procedure.

Once the pre-transplant evaluation is successfully completed, the patient is placed on the transplant waiting list in order to await the availability of a suitable donor organ. The complexities of organ allocation highlight the difficulty of the transplantation procedure by taking into account variables such organ compatibility, the severity of the patient's disease, and geographic proximity. Following the discovery of a suitable donor organ, the surgical transplantation occurs, which is the last step in a thorough process that aims to improve the recipient's overall prognosis and restore their liver function.

Managing liver transplantation requires the participation of various viewpoints, each of which is essential to the effective implementation of this intricate procedure. As far as healthcare providers are concerned, the focus is on making sure that multidisciplinary teams—which include hepatologists, transplant surgeons, transplant coordinators, and other medical professionals—coordinate seamlessly. Patients awaiting transplantation must also be included in this process, as they must negotiate the psychological and physical challenges of waiting for a new organ as well as the uncertainties around organ availability and the upcoming surgery.

Another aspect of liver transplantation is the involvement of living donors, who selflessly donate a portion of their healthy liver to a recipient who is in need of saving their own life. Through illuminating these diverse viewpoints, a thorough comprehension of the cooperative character of liver transplantation surfaced, highlighting the interdependence of parties involved in attaining favourable transplant results.

The utilisation of factual information and data based on evidence is crucial in supporting liver transplantation's efficacy and safety as the ultimate treatment for end-stage liver disease. For example, research has shown that liver transplantation dramatically improves long-term survival rates for patients with severe cirrhosis, providing a large survival benefit. Citing particular study findings gives the prescription for transplantation as the final intervention a solid empirical foundation and clarifies the significant impact of this surgery on patient outcomes.

Additionally, by including data on graft survival rates, long-term results, and post-transplant problems, readers are given a quantitative understanding of the efficacy of liver transplantation as a therapeutic approach. Through the integration of data and facts, anyone navigating the intricacies of liver transplantation can acquire a thorough comprehension of the evidence bolstering this revolutionary operation.

The field of liver transplantation involves many technical words and ideas that patients and caregivers may find difficult to understand. For example, the complexities of immunosuppressive treatment, which tries to stop organ rejection after transplantation, require a precise explanation of the ideas behind these drugs and how they affect the immune system of the recipient. Simplifying these complicated phrases makes it easier for a wider audience to understand the reasoning behind post-transplant pharmaceutical regimens, enabling them to take an active role in their treatment after transplant.

Furthermore, explaining terms associated with the surgical process, organ matching, and post-transplant monitoring helps patients grasp the complexities of liver transplantation. Clear explanations of these technical words enable those considering transplantation to make well-informed decisions and actively participate in their post-transplant care, both of which improve the likelihood of a successful transplant.

In summary, navigating the liver transplantation process is a complex journey that includes rigorous selection criteria, thorough evaluation processes, surgical transplantation, and extensive post-transplant care. Through a thorough explanation of the concepts, the inclusion of data and facts, the exploration of various perspectives, the clarification of complex terms, the emphasis on important takeaways, and a thorough exploration of the data, readers are able to gain a deeper understanding of the complexities related to liver transplantation. In the end, this information empowers people to understand and handle the complexities of liver transplantation, leading to the best possible outcomes in the treatment of severe cirrhosis.

Emerging Therapies

The treatment of cirrhosis has undergone a dynamic evolution marked by an ongoing search for new therapeutic approaches to slow the course of the illness, enhance patient outcomes, and meet unmet clinical demands. Novel approaches to the treatment of cirrhosis include a wide range of interventions, including pharmaceutical treatments, surgical techniques, and innovative research projects. With a focus on the historical roots, current developments, and potential future directions that together influence the paradigm of cirrhosis treatment, this chapter attempts to present a thorough overview of the field of new therapeutics in cirrhosis management.

Emerging therapeutics for the management of cirrhosis have their roots in the early research endeavours of physicians and medical researchers who aimed to broaden the range of therapeutic options beyond traditional methods. Historical narratives demonstrate the progressive transition from reactive symptom care to an active search for therapeutic approaches aimed at addressing the underlying pathophysiological causes of cirrhosis. A significant turning point in the history of cirrhosis care was the introduction of liver transplantation as the only effective treatment for end-stage cirrhosis. This led to a change in the way that advanced liver disease is approached.

The development of new treatments for the treatment of cirrhosis is dotted with significant turning points that have altered the direction of clinical practise and research. The discovery of antifibrotic drugs that may reduce hepatic fibrosis, the development of minimally invasive methods for controlling portal hypertension, and the clarification of the complex relationship between the gut microbiota and the pathophysiology of cirrhosis are important historical developments. Personalized care of cirrhosis has advanced significantly with the advent of precision medicine approaches that use genetic and molecular analysis to customise therapeutic therapies.

Visual aids that improve comprehension of the complex ideas underlying new treatments in cirrhosis management include histopathological pictures that show the histological alterations in cirrhotic liver tissue, schematic representations of novel therapeutic targets, and graphical illustrations that clarify the mechanisms of action of emerging pharmacological agents. Through the use of visual aids, readers are able to obtain a thorough visual understanding of the scientific and clinical elements of these novel therapeutic approaches, leading to a more profound understanding of their potential utility in the treatment of cirrhosis.

Diverse cultural and regional contexts have not experienced the development of emergent medicines in cirrhosis management in the same way, leading to noteworthy differences in the uptake and application of new strategies. The necessity for fair diffusion of breakthroughs in cirrhosis management is underscored by the variations in access to and utilisation of novel medications caused by sociocultural variables, healthcare infrastructure variability, and economic inequities. Additionally, the adoption and integration of innovative therapeutic modalities have been influenced by cultural beliefs and practises related to disease management; hence, a comprehensive understanding of cultural and regional variances in the implementation of developing therapies is necessary.

Modern interpretations and modifications of novel treatments for cirrhosis involve the incorporation of state-of-the-art technologies, such as machine learning and artificial intelligence, to support early disease identification, risk assessment, and treatment planning. Furthermore, the coming together of hepatologists, pharmacologists, geneticists, and bioinformaticians in multidisciplinary collaborations has sparked the creation of novel therapeutic platforms and opened the door for precision-targeted interventions catered to the distinct molecular signatures of individual cirrhotic patients. Furthermore, the rapidly developing field of regenerative medicine presents opportunities for the creation of cutting-edge treatment approaches targeted at liver tissue regeneration and cirrhosis-related functional restoration.

The field of developing treatments for managing cirrhosis is not without difficulties, disagreements, and significant turning points that have influenced the course of clinical advancement. The challenges include the need to strike a balance between the need to rigorously evaluate safety and efficacy profiles and the imperative of translating preclinical research findings into clinical applications as quickly as possible, all while ensuring that emerging therapies adhere to the highest standards of patient care. The complexity of navigating the landscape of developing therapeutics in cirrhosis management is further highlighted by debates over the cost-effectiveness of innovative therapy, ethical issues in research conduct, and the unexpected consequences of therapeutic approaches. A new era in the management of cirrhosis has been brought about by pivotal moments such as the realisation that the gut-liver axis is a central nexus in the pathogenesis of cirrhosis and the paradigm shift towards individualised therapeutic strategies. These events have brought about transformative changes in the way emerging therapies are conceptualised and applied.

To sum up, investigating novel treatments for cirrhosis management reveals a rich tapestry of clinical creativity, scientific advancement, and translational promise that will have a significant impact on how cirrhosis is treated in the future. This chapter aims to provide readers with a thorough understanding of the dynamic evolution of therapeutic strategies in the management of cirrhosis by tracing the historical roots, explaining current advancements, and outlining potential future directions. It also hopes to foster an appreciation for the complex interactions that exist between scientific discovery and clinical application in the pursuit of the best possible patient outcomes.

Understanding Surgery Options

Surgical procedures are essential to the overall therapy of cirrhosis because they provide a variety of alternatives for addressing complications and enhancing patient outcomes. The objective of this chapter is to assess the surgical options available for managing complications from cirrhosis, including a thorough examination of their parallels, divergences, and wider implications within the framework of managing cirrhosis.

The issues included in this review include surgical procedures that are frequently used to treat difficulties arising from cirrhosis, such as liver transplantation, surgical shunts, and hepatic resection. These operations are clinically significant in that they address a wide range of problems related to cirrhosis, from hepatocellular cancer to portal hypertension. In order to optimise results for patients with cirrhosis and to customise the therapeutic approach to meet the specific needs of each patient, it is imperative to comprehend the subtleties of each surgical intervention.

The goal of comparing surgical techniques for managing cirrhosis is to clarify the unique characteristics and therapeutic possibilities of each approach, which will help physicians make better decisions and provide better care for their patients. This analysis attempts to offer insights into the best choice and implementation of surgical procedures in the setting of cirrhosis complications by outlining the distinctive characteristics and clinical implications of these surgical modalities.

The benchmarks used for comparison include each surgical procedure's efficacy, safety profile, indications, contraindications, and long-term results. Additionally, factors including the patient's candidacy, the severity of the disease, and the underlying cause of the cirrhosis are important factors to take into account while assessing all available surgical options for the therapy of cirrhosis.

The goal of both surgical shunts and liver transplantation is to treat portal hypertension-related problems in cirrhotic patients. Through different methods, the two therapies seek to mitigate the hemodynamic changes and lower the risk of variceal haemorrhage. While surgical shunts directly divert blood flow to lower elevated portal pressure, liver transplantation provides a permanent solution for the underlying liver illness while managing portal hypertension. On the other hand, hepatic resection is mainly recommended for specific individuals who have cirrhosis-related hepatocellular carcinoma and want to remove the tumour while leaving the functional hepatic parenchyma intact.

There are several key differences between hepatic resection, surgical shunts, and liver transplantation. These include the extent of their therapeutic uses, degree of invasiveness, long-term effects, and suitability for different clinical situations. As the last resort for treating end-stage liver disease, liver transplantation presents the possibility of curing cirrhosis and all of its complications completely. However, it also comes with a number of challenges, including the need for careful patient selection, ongoing immunosuppression, and the problem of organ scarcity. Surgical shunts, on the other hand, offer a palliative approach to portal hypertension and provide rapid hemodynamic relief. However, they come with risks, including the possibility of encephalopathy, shunt dysfunction, and disease progression in the native liver. Hepatic resection has the potential to be curative for hepatocellular carcinoma; nevertheless, it is limited by the need for sufficient hepatic reserves, the danger of decompensation following surgery, and the possibility of disease recurrence.

The intricate ideas behind each surgical treatment can be made easier to understand by using visual aids such schematics of the hemodynamic changes in cirrhosis, anatomical drawings of surgical shunts, and graphical representations of the indications for hepatic resection. Visual aids promote a fuller grasp of these interventions' involvement in managing cirrhosis by improving the reader's comprehension of the subtleties and clinical implications of these treatments.

A comparative study of surgical techniques used in the management of cirrhosis demonstrates the various therapeutic environments provided by hepatic resection, surgical shunts, and liver transplantation, each of which is designed to address particular clinical scenarios and complications in patients with cirrhosis. The analysis provided valuable insights that highlight the need of customised treatment plans, careful patient selection, and interdisciplinary teamwork in maximising surgical outcomes for cirrhosis patients.

This comparison approach is still relevant today because it may be applied to the clinical setting to help physicians make decisions about surgery for patients with cirrhosis. The evaluation's conclusions are still relevant today given the changes in perioperative care, surgical procedures, and the range of treatment choices available for complications related to cirrhosis.

Finally, a range of therapeutic modalities with unique characteristics, clinical implications, and therapeutic potentials are revealed by evaluating surgical possibilities in the therapy of cirrhosis. This analysis attempts to enhance knowledge of surgical procedures in the setting of cirrhosis by outlining their parallels, distinctions, and wider consequences. It also fosters an appreciation of the complex surgical care landscape in cirrhotic patients.

Managing Complications

A wide range of problems are frequently associated with cirrhosis, a chronic and progressive liver disease that has a substantial impact on patient outcomes. Hepatic encephalopathy, ascites, variceal haemorrhage, and hepatorenal syndrome are among the consequences that make managing cirrhotic patients extremely difficult. Comprehending and proficiently handling these consequences is vital in order to alleviate their deleterious impact on the general well-being and standard of living of cirrhosis patients.

A major obstacle in the treatment of cirrhosis is the development of hepatic encephalopathy, a complicated neuropsychiatric condition resulting from liver failure and portosystemic shunting. A range of cognitive and motor abnormalities, from mild attention and mood disorders to severe disorientation, stupor, and coma, are indicative of hepatic encephalopathy. If treatment for this illness is not received, there is a significant risk of morbidity and mortality in addition to the impairment of everyday activities and cognitive function in patients.

Ineffective management of hepatic encephalopathy can result in a deterioration of the patient's general cognitive function, which will affect their capacity to perform daily activities and continue participating in social and professional activities. Furthermore, severe or recurrent bouts of hepatic encephalopathy may require frequent hospital stays, which will raise the cost of healthcare and lower the standard of living for the patient and their carers. Furthermore, the severity of uncontrolled hepatic encephalopathy is further exacerbated by the likelihood of complications such as sepsis and aspiration pneumonia.

Hepatic encephalopathy is treated with a multimodal strategy that targets precipitating causes, improves ammonia clearance, and lowers ammonia generation. The mainstays of managing hepatic encephalopathy include pharmacological therapies, dietary changes, and the identification and treatment of triggering causes. Optimizing patient outcomes requires individualised treatment regimens that are specific to the degree and underlying causes of hepatic encephalopathy.

Agents that target the gut microbiota and lessen ammonia generation and absorption, such as lactulose, rifaximin, and non-absorbable disaccharides, are used in the pharmacological therapy of hepatic encephalopathy. Dietary changes that promote liver function and reduce the risk of hepatic encephalopathy include protein limitation and the use of branched-chain amino acid supplements. To further prevent the recurrence of hepatic encephalopathy, precipitating events like gastrointestinal bleeding, infections, and electrolyte abnormalities must be identified and treated.

Lactulose and rifaximin have been shown in numerous studies to be effective in lessening the frequency and severity of episodes of hepatic encephalopathy, which in turn improves cognitive function and quality of life in patients with cirrhosis. Furthermore, nutritional therapies targeting the regulation of ammonia metabolism and enhancement of liver function have demonstrated encouraging results in the treatment of hepatic encephalopathy. The management of hepatic encephalopathy can be made more manageable and patient outcomes can be improved by healthcare practitioners by employing a thorough and customised approach.

Although the cornerstones of managing hepatic encephalopathy are pharmaceutical and nutritional measures, newer approaches to treating this problem include ammonia-lowering medications and microbiota modification. Moreover, further investigation into the pathophysiology of hepatic encephalopathy and the roles played by inflammation and oxidative stress may provide new targets for treatment in the future.

In summary, stopping the course of this crippling consequence and enhancing patient outcomes depend critically on the appropriate therapy of hepatic encephalopathy in cirrhotic patients. Healthcare professionals can lessen the effects of hepatic encephalopathy and improve the quality of life for people with cirrhosis by putting into practise a thorough and customised strategy that incorporates pharmacological, nutritional, and precipitating factor-targeted therapies.

Interventional Radiology

Interventional Radiology in the Management of Cirrhosis

Because of its complexity and variety, cirrhosis is a disease that can be difficult to control and frequently requires a multidisciplinary approach to treat its many problems. The importance of interventional radiology, a specialisation of radiology that focuses on using minimally invasive techniques to diagnose and treat disorders within the body, is one of the most important aspects of managing cirrhosis. The use of interventional radiology techniques in the care of cirrhosis includes a broad range of operations intended to address problems like vascular anomalies, hepatic cancers, and portal hypertension. The purpose of this chapter is to clarify the critical role that interventional radiology plays in the all-encompassing care of cirrhosis by offering a thorough examination of its uses, results, and possible future developments.

The medical profession known as interventional radiology, or IR, uses image-guided minimally invasive treatments to diagnose and treat disorders. By providing minimally invasive, frequently effective, and less risky alternatives to established surgical methods, interventional radiology plays a critical role in managing problems associated with cirrhosis, including portal hypertension, hepatocellular carcinoma, and vascular anomalies.

A wide variety of treatments fall under the umbrella of interventional radiology, such as image-guided biopsies, embolization, percutaneous interventions, and angiography. These methods offer patients alternatives to surgery and lengthier recovery times by diagnosing and treating a range of diseases.

The treatment of portal hypertension, a frequent cirrhosis consequence brought on by increased resistance to portal blood flow, is a crucial component of interventional radiology in the management of cirrhosis. Ascites, hepatic encephalopathy, and varices are all conditions that are exacerbated by portal hypertension and have a major negative effect on patient outcomes. Interventional radiologists use methods such creating a transjugular intrahepatic portosystemic shunt (TIPS) to lessen the consequences of portal hypertension and lower the risk of refractory ascites and variceal haemorrhage.

Moreover, hepatocellular carcinoma (HCC), the most prevalent primary liver cancer, is diagnosed, staged, and treated in large part thanks to interventional radiology. Minimally invasive methods for treating HCC are provided by image-guided techniques such as radiofrequency ablation (RFA) and transcatheter arterial chemoembolization (TACE), which are frequently used in patients whose severe disease prevents them from undergoing surgical resection.

Vascular anomalies in cirrhotic patients are managed using interventional radiology procedures together with hepatic malignancies and portal hypertension. This covers the therapy of issues associated with liver transplantation, such as hepatic artery thrombosis and biliary strictures, as well as the treatment of vascular abnormalities like portosystemic shunts.

With the advent of angiography in the middle of the 20th century and the subsequent development of less invasive procedures, interventional radiology came into being. Significant developments in imaging technology, procedural instruments, and treatment modalities have been made in interventional radiology over the years, broadening its application and increasing its effectiveness in the treatment of a variety of illnesses, including those linked to cirrhosis.

As a key player in the interdisciplinary management of cirrhosis, interventional radiology works together with hepatologists, transplant surgeons, oncologists, and other experts to offer patients with cirrhosis complete care. Interventional radiology improves patient outcomes and quality of life while lowering procedure risks and recovery times by providing minimally invasive options to manage diverse complications of cirrhosis.

One noteworthy use of interventional radiology in the treatment of cirrhosis is the application of TIPS to the control of variceal haemorrhage and refractory ascites. TIPS formation is a procedure that lowers portal pressure and improves portal hypertension symptoms by implanting a stent inside the liver to form a shunt between the portal and hepatic veins. For cirrhotic patients experiencing these problems, this technique has been effective in managing refractory ascites and minimising variceal rebleeding, providing a crucial therapeutic option.

Interventional radiology methods like TACE and RFA have completely changed the therapy options available to patients with incurable hepatocellular carcinoma. In TACE, the hepatic artery is used to deliver chemotherapy drugs to the tumour selectively. The tumor's blood supply is then cut off by embolization. In contrast, RFA uses heat radiation to destroy the tumour tissue, providing a treatment for those with minor HCC lesions. Patients who are not candidates for surgical resection now have more therapeutic choices for treating HCC thanks to these minimally invasive techniques.

The idea that interventional radiology is only a diagnostic specialism, ignoring its significant contributions to therapeutic interventions, is a prevalent misperception about the field. Although interventional radiologists are essential to diagnostic imaging, their knowledge goes well beyond interpretation of imaging results. They are skilled in a variety of minimally invasive procedures that can significantly improve patient care in a number of medical specialties, including the management of cirrhosis.

To sum up, interventional radiology provides minimally invasive approaches to treat problems such portal hypertension, hepatocellular carcinoma, and vascular anomalies, making it an essential part of the overall care of cirrhosis. Interventional radiologists apply minimally invasive procedures and advanced imaging techniques to improve patient outcomes, improve the quality of life for patients with cirrhosis, and support a multidisciplinary approach to managing the disease. The role of interventional radiology in managing cirrhosis is set to change as technology and procedural knowledge continue to progress. This will enhance the treatment provided to patients with this complicated illness by broadening their therapeutic options and enhancing their overall quality of life.

The Role of Clinical Trials

Clinical trials are essential for expanding our understanding of medicine and enhancing patient care for a variety of diseases, including cirrhosis. The field of cirrhosis management may change as a result of the thorough and methodical examination of novel therapies, therapeutic approaches, and diagnostic technologies through clinical trials. In order to clarify the significance of evidence-based research in determining the standard of care for cirrhotic patients, this chapter will examine the effects of clinical trials on the treatment of cirrhosis.

Engaging in clinical trials has a substantial impact on the management of cirrhosis by promoting innovation in cirrhosis care, evaluating new therapies, and developing evidence-based guidelines.

The ability to evaluate the safety and effectiveness of novel therapy modalities forms the cornerstone of clinical trials in the management of cirrhosis. Through phases of clinical trials, investigational medications, techniques, and interventions are rigorously evaluated to provide vital information about their effects on patients with cirrhosis. Trials assessing new medications, for example, to treat portal hypertension, a common cirrhosis consequence, provide important information about the possible advantages and disadvantages of these treatments, influencing the range of treatment options that patients and clinicians can choose from.

A platform for clarifying the best management approaches for cirrhotic consequences is provided by clinical trials. Comparative trials are a useful tool for researchers to evaluate the efficacy of alternative treatment approaches. For example, researchers might compare different interventional procedures for controlling portal hypertension or evaluate different surgical techniques for hepatic malignancies. Critical evidence from these trials helps doctors make well-informed decisions that are customised to the unique needs of patients with cirrhosis, improving their care and results.

Additionally, clinical trials aid in the clarification of risk stratification instruments and prognostic markers in cirrhosis. Trials offer important information for improving risk assessment models and individualised treatment algorithms, which in turn improves the accuracy and effectiveness of cirrhosis management. These models are refined by examining the effects of particular biomarkers, imaging modalities, or genetic factors on disease progression and treatment response.

Clinical trials have a significant influence on the care of cirrhosis; however, there are obstacles and restrictions related to study participation and result interpretation. Trials face substantial challenges in patient recruitment and retention, which frequently result in sample biases and restrict the applicability of findings to larger cirrhotic populations. The intricacy of converting trial findings into clinical practise is further highlighted by the interpretation of trial data, which requires careful evaluation of potential confounders, differences in patient characteristics, and the dynamic nature of cirrhosis pathophysiology.

Acknowledging the difficulties that come with conducting clinical trials, it is important to remember that efforts to improve trial design, patient involvement, and data analysis are always changing in an attempt to lessen these constraints. Concerns about sample representativeness and result generalizability are being addressed by innovations in trial techniques, such as adaptive trial designs and real-world evidence integration, which are broadening the scope and robustness of trial findings. Additionally, a thorough and patient-centered approach to trial conduct and interpretation is fostered by the cooperation of researchers, regulatory agencies, and patient advocacy groups; this strengthens the validity and application of trial outcomes to cirrhosis management in the real world.

Clinical trials are essential for assessing behavioural therapies, lifestyle changes, and integrated care models for patients with cirrhosis, in addition to medicinal and diagnostic research. Trials evaluating the effects of fitness programmes, dietary changes, and psychological support on the course of cirrhosis contribute to the comprehensive therapy of the illness, highlighting the multifaceted approach to cirrhosis care that is backed by research with solid evidence.

To sum up, clinical trials have a broad and diverse influence on the management of cirrhosis. They include the assessment of new therapies, the improvement of treatment algorithms, and the development of individualised care plans. Even though there are still issues with trial conduct and interpretation, ongoing developments in trial methodology and cooperative approaches show promise for improving the trial findings' relevance and applicability to the intricate world of managing cirrhosis. The significance of clinical trials in developing evidence-based guidelines and promoting innovation is crucial in improving the care and outcomes of those living with cirrhosis, and this role will only grow as the field of cirrhosis research advances.

Holistic Health Strategies

The Power of Nutrition

This chapter aims to emphasise the critical role that diet plays in maintaining liver health and controlling cirrhosis. Readers will have a thorough understanding of how a customised diet can improve liver function and help treat cirrhosis by the end of this chapter.

In order to properly appreciate the ideas covered in this chapter, readers need be familiar with the pathophysiology of cirrhosis and liver function. It will also be helpful to have access to reliable dietary information sources and management guidelines for cirrhosis.

We will examine the complex relationship between nutrition and liver health in this chapter, as well as the effects of dietary patterns, macronutrients, and micronutrients on the development of cirrhosis. Additionally, we will go over the significance of customised meal plans and the possible advantages of nutritional supplementation for individuals with cirrhosis.

Break down each part of the process in detail.

1. Understanding the Role of Nutrition in Cirrhosis Management:

Understanding the basic function that nutrition plays in liver health and illness is the first step. We will discuss the idea of hepatic encephalopathy, how diet affects liver function, and how malnutrition affects the course of cirrhosis.

2. Tailoring the Diet to Support Liver Health:

This section will concentrate on the particular dietary adjustments required to maintain liver health in people with cirrhosis. We will go over the value of maintaining an appropriate caloric intake, the role of protein restriction in hepatic encephalopathy, and the importance of macronutrient balance.

3. Nutritional Strategies for Managing Complications of Cirrhosis:

We shall discuss nutritional treatment of typical cirrhosis problems here, including sarcopenia, hepatic encephalopathy, and ascites. We will discuss the application of branched-chain amino acids, the function of sodium restriction, and the possible advantages of specific dietary formulas.

4. The Impact of Micronutrients and Antioxidants:

The significance of antioxidants and micronutrients in the treatment of cirrhosis will be emphasised in this section. We'll talk about how vitamins, minerals, and phytochemicals help the body fight oxidative stress, boost the immune system, and encourage the regeneration of the liver.

Practical Advice: - Stress the value of including nutrient-dense foods and a diverse diet.

- Promote routine dietary and laboratory tests and assessments of nutritional status.

- Promote the use of a certified dietitian or other nutrition specialist in the treatment of cirrhosis.

- Cautionary Advice: - Advise against consuming large amounts of alcohol and the possible interaction between some drugs and food ingredients.

Emphasize the necessity of tailored dietary guidelines depending on the particular cause and degree of cirrhosis.

Describe how to verify successful completion.

Successful completion of this chapter will be demonstrated by the reader's ability to outline a personalised dietary plan for cirrhotic individuals, identify potential nutritional interventions for managing complications related to cirrhosis, and demonstrate a thorough understanding of the relationship between nutrition and cirrhosis management.

Readers are advised to see medical professionals who specialise in liver disease and nutrition if they encounter difficulties implementing a customised diet or interpreting nutritional recommendations.

To sum up, this chapter provides a solid framework for understanding how important diet is for maintaining liver function and treating cirrhosis. Through the adoption of the concepts and tactics delineated in this section, readers will possess enhanced abilities to maximise their nutritional state and constructively influence the advancement of cirrhosis.

Herbal Allies

The study of herbs and supplements for liver support has attracted a lot of interest in the field of cirrhosis therapy. There has been discussion and interest in the possibility of herbal allies to support liver health and supplement conventional treatments. In order to better understand herbal treatments and nutritional supplements, this chapter will examine their efficacy, safety, and possible application in the treatment of cirrhosis. We seek to offer a thorough grasp of herbal allies' effects on liver function and their applicability in the full treatment of cirrhosis by investigating the claims and data surrounding them.

The main assertion that is being investigated is the possible effectiveness of dietary supplements and herbal treatments in promoting liver health and controlling problems associated with cirrhosis. The proposal suggests that some herbs and supplements have the potential to mitigate liver damage and alleviate cirrhotic conditions due to their hepatoprotective, antioxidant, and anti-inflammatory qualities.

We start by looking at the main data that backs up the use of herbal allies in the treatment of cirrhosis in order to validate the claim. A number of plants and supplements, such as milk thistle, turmeric, and artichoke extract, have been investigated for their possible hepatoprotective properties. These organic substances have proven to be antioxidants, have anti-fibrotic effects, and have the capacity to alter inflammatory pathways—all of which are important for maintaining liver function and managing cirrhosis.

Originating from the Silybum marianum plant, milk thistle has arguably been studied more than any other herb when it comes to liver health. Through a variety of methods, including the control of hepatic stellate cell activity, the decrease of oxidative stress, and the inhibition of pro-inflammatory pathways, the active ingredient, silymarin, has been demonstrated to display hepatoprotective properties. Research has indicated that it may be useful in reducing liver fibrosis and improving liver function in individuals with cirrhosis.

Similarly, turmeric's anti-inflammatory and antioxidant qualities have drawn interest because it contains the bioactive component curcumin. Research has been done on curcumin's ability to reduce liver damage, alter immunological responses, and stop liver fibrosis from getting worse. These results offer a compelling possibility for adding supplements containing curcumin, or turmeric, to cirrhosis treatment regimens.

The hepatoprotective efficacy of artichoke extract, which is enhanced with bioactive substances including cynarin and derivatives of caffeic acid, has also been investigated. Studies have demonstrated its function in augmenting bile flow, encouraging liver detoxification, and exhibiting antioxidant properties. These mechanisms may be important to consider while managing issues associated with cirrhosis, especially when it comes to managing cholestasis and bolstering hepatic metabolism.

Even in the face of overwhelming evidence that suggests herbal allies are effective, it is important to recognise the opposing data and arguments to their stated advantages. Over the safety and dependability of herbal preparations in clinical practise, there are legitimate concerns due to scepticism regarding standardisation, variability in bioavailability, and potential herb-drug interactions. Furthermore, the absence of reliable clinical trials and inconsistent study results for several herbal medicines highlight the need for caution when interpreting their therapeutic potential.

To ensure reproducibility and consistency in their composition in response to the counter-evidence, it is critical to stress the need of standardised herbal extracts and quality control procedures. Strict research procedures, such as systematic reviews and randomised controlled trials, are essential for verifying the safety and effectiveness of herbal remedies in the treatment of cirrhosis. In order to reduce any hazards and potential interactions with conventional pharmaceuticals, the integration of herbal therapies should be done so cautiously and after consulting with healthcare professionals.

Emerging data bolsters the assertion by pointing to the possible advantages of various herbal companions, including schisandra, licorice root, and dandelion, in enhancing liver health and treating symptoms associated with cirrhosis. These plants have a variety of pharmacological characteristics, such as hepatoprotective, immunomodulatory, and anti-inflammatory actions, that should be investigated in relation to the treatment of cirrhosis. The spectrum of natural therapies for cirrhosis can be expanded by looking into the therapeutic potential of these herbal allies in clinical settings, as supported by preliminary research and preclinical evidence.

To sum up, research into nutritional supplements and herbal allies for liver support is a promising path toward improving the overall treatment of cirrhosis. Despite the encouraging evidence for their effectiveness, care must be taken when integrating them to ensure that high standards are met, robust research validation is done, and clinical decision-making is well-informed. In order to fully realise the benefits of herbal medicines and supplements as supplementary therapy in the management of cirrhosis, further research and critical evaluation are required, all the while ensuring patient safety and wellbeing.

Mind-Body Connections

A noteworthy case study takes place in the clinical environment of our cirrhosis management programme, illuminating the complex interactions between psychological and emotional health activities and how they affect the overall treatment of cirrhosis. The main character of the scenario is Mr. Jacobson, a 52-year-old man with non-alcoholic fatty liver disease (NAFLD)-related severe cirrhosis who presents with crippling exhaustion, mental anguish, and a decreased quality of life. We explore his path and uncover the obstacles, approaches, and results that lead to a better comprehension of the mind-body relationships in the treatment of cirrhosis.

The condition of severe cirrhosis presented a difficult reality to Mr. Jacobson, a former business executive. This illness not only caused physical difficulties but also caused intense emotional and psychological distress. In order to treat the many aspects of his condition, his multidisciplinary care team—which included hepatologists, nutritionists, physical therapists, and mental health specialists—worked together to create a thorough management plan that encompassed holistic wellness principles.

The central issue in Mr. Jacobson's case was the complex network of problems resulting from the mutually reinforcing relationship between his physical illness and the consequences it had for his mental and emotional health. He faced significant challenges to his overall quality of life due to his chronic exhaustion, the distress of receiving a life-altering diagnosis, and the loss of vitality, which called for a more nuanced approach than was typically provided by conventional medical interventions.

The management method included a multimodal approach that combined traditional medical care with techniques for psychological and emotional well-being. Mr. Jacobson began receiving individualised counselling sessions designed to help him deal with the psychological effects of his diagnosis, build resilience, and develop coping skills to help him deal with the challenges of having cirrhosis. In order to lessen psychological suffering and improve his emotional balance, mindfulness-based stress reduction techniques, relaxation exercises, and guided imagery were also included.

Moreover, the incorporation of lifestyle modifications, such as customised exercise programmes and nutritional alterations, was crucial in strengthening his mental and physical resilience. By using the positive feedback loop that is created between physical activity and emotional well-being, Mr. Jacobson was able to take control of his health journey and regain a sense of agency.

The dramatic results of this integrated method extended beyond the confines of conventional medical measures to include aspects of psychological well-being and emotional vigour. Mr. Jacobson reported feeling more emotionally stable and resilient, as well as a noticeable decrease in his overall sensation of exhaustion. He had a noticeable change in perspective as a result of his involvement with the holistic management plan, which gave him more agency and empowerment in overcoming the challenges presented by his illness.

Validated instruments assessing emotional well-being, fatigue severity, and overall psychological adjustment showed increases in his quality of life parameters, according to quantitative assessments. The objective measures of advancement aligned with Mr. Jacobson's subjective feelings, highlighting the transforming effect of incorporating mind-body links in the management of cirrhosis.

The case of Mr. Jacobson offers priceless insights into the profoundly beneficial relationship between holistic cirrhosis management and psychological and emotional wellbeing measures. It highlights the necessity of understanding the interconnectedness of mental and physical health and the need for an all-encompassing strategy that goes beyond traditional medical paradigms. In addition, the instance prompts contemplation of the possible foundations of mind-body links as stimulants for fortitude, self-determination, and enhanced therapeutic results in the treatment of cirrhosis.

An integrated mind-body approach would have a demonstrable effect on Mr. Jacobson's overall well-being if there were visuals that showed the progression of his quality of life metrics, tiredness severity ratings, and emotional well-being assessments.

Mr. Jacobson's example represents a microcosm of the complex storey that underlies the incorporation of mind-body links in the treatment of cirrhosis. It emphasises how important it is to recognise the unbreakable connection between mental and physical health, and it pushes for a paradigm change that includes holistic wellness ideas as essential components of total health care. The case provides a powerful example of the transforming power of incorporating psychological and emotional wellness practises into the larger framework of cirrhosis management, so creating a paradigm of care that goes beyond the conventional bounds of medical intervention.

A crucial query arises as we explore the complex web of mind-body relationships in the management of cirrhosis: How can the incorporation of psychological and emotional wellness practises be further leveraged to reshape the terrain of all-encompassing care for people managing the complexities of cirrhosis? This question invites us to explore the rich possibilities of mind-body relationships as drivers of empowerment, resilience, and overall health in the context of managing cirrhosis.

Movement as Medicine

In the complicated web of managing cirrhosis, physical exercise plays a crucial role as a cornerstone of the holistic approach to addressing the various aspects of this multifaceted disorder. When it comes to cirrhosis, movement as medicine goes beyond traditional models of physical therapy and becomes extremely important for bolstering not just the physical but also the mental and emotional health of those coping with the intricacies of this long-term illness.

The incorporation of physical exercise as a therapeutic modality in the therapy of cirrhosis is woven throughout the holistic care framework, embracing a range of therapies that beyond the boundaries of traditional medical care. Movement and medicine work in unison to provide a storey that goes beyond the confines of conventional thinking and helps people grasp the profoundly positive effects of physical activity as part of a comprehensive care plan for cirrhosis patients.

The core principle of including physical exercise into the management of cirrhosis stems from its complex effects on an individual's psychological, emotional, and physiological aspects. Exercise that is customised to meet the specific requirements and abilities of people with cirrhosis produces a range of advantages that go beyond the scope of conventional therapy, including increases in muscle strength, stamina, and functional ability. Moreover, the significant effects of physical activity extend beyond the boundaries of the physiological domain and penetrate the psychological and emotional domains by promoting emotional balance, empowerment, and a sense of action.

The complexities of cirrhosis offer a patchwork of difficulties that impair the patient's physical and mental health, including exhaustion, deconditioning of the musculoskeletal system, and reduced functional ability. These complex aspects are addressed by incorporating physical activity as a cornerstone of therapy in the management of cirrhosis. This approach creates a paradigm of care that embraces the transformative power of movement as medicine and goes beyond the limitations of traditional medical interventions.

Examine Ms. Rodriguez's situation. She is a 45-year-old woman who is dealing with the consequences of severe cirrhosis brought on by persistent hepatitis C. Her entire quality of life was severely hampered by the burden of her disease, which took the shape of crippling weariness, musculoskeletal deconditioning, and a discernible decline in her functional ability. The implementation of a customised fitness programme, consisting of a range of activities catered to her individual requirements and abilities, resulted in a significant improvement in her physical toughness, psychological stability, and general standard of living.

In addition, the storey of Mr. Patel, a 58-year-old man managing the complications of cirrhosis due to alcoholic liver disease, provides evidence of the transforming power of exercise in the comprehensive treatment of cirrhosis. The incorporation of structured exercise programmes, which included a combination of resistance, aerobic, and flexibility exercises, strengthened his physical resilience and led to a noticeable improvement in his emotional stability, which in turn produced a noticeable change in his perspective and general quality of life.

The incorporation of physical activity as a fundamental component in managing cirrhosis spans a variety of viewpoints that go beyond the boundaries of conventional rehabilitation models. From the perspective of the person living with cirrhosis, exercise acts as a trigger, promoting emotional balance, empowerment, and a sense of agency in overcoming the challenges associated with this long-term illness. Beyond the confines of traditional medical interventions, the integration of physical activity as a therapeutic modality fosters a paradigm of care that embraces the profound symbiosis between movement and medicine in the continuum of cirrhosis management, as seen through the eyes of the multidisciplinary care team.

A substantial body of research, including empirical data and clinical studies, supports the integration of physical activity as a therapeutic cornerstone in the management of cirrhosis. These studies highlight the multifaceted impact of physical activity on an individual's physiological, emotional, and psychological dimensions. Research from both clinical trials and long-term research has demonstrated how beneficial physical activity is for people with cirrhosis in terms of reducing fatigue, strengthening musculoskeletal resilience, and improving their overall quality of life. Moreover, the scientific evidence highlights the range of advantages that physical activity produces, which extend beyond the physiological domain to include enhancements in psychological balance, emotional stability, and adaptability to the intricacies of cirrhosis.

Incorporating physical activity as a therapeutic modality into the therapy of cirrhosis involves a range of interventions that are customised to meet the specific requirements and abilities of those living with this chronic illness. When viewed through the lens of rehabilitation, physical activity transcends traditional boundaries and includes a combination of resistance, aerobic, and flexibility activities designed to strengthen physiological resilience, improve musculoskeletal endurance, and promote emotional balance. Furthermore, the subtleties of physical activity in managing cirrhosis extend to emotional and psychological health, promoting a strong sense of agency, empowerment, and emotional balance in negotiating the complexity of this long-term condition.

The storey of using physical exercise as a cornerstone of therapy in the management of cirrhosis reveals a profound awareness of the healing power of movement as medicine in the continuum of care for patients coping with this chronic illness. The incorporation of customised exercise programmes that include a range of interventions results in a noticeable change in the psychological, emotional, and physiological aspects of the person, highlighting the comprehensive role that physical activity plays in promoting emotional stability, resilience, and general well-being. Throughout the complex journey of managing cirrhosis, the therapeutic potential of physical activity invites us to adopt a care paradigm that goes beyond the boundaries of conventional rehabilitation. This approach leverages movement's transformative power as medicine within the continuum of cirrhosis management.

Detoxification Techniques

Detoxification procedures are an essential part of the overall care of cirrhosis because they provide a range of safe and efficient ways to support the body's natural detoxification processes. The incorporation of these methods extends beyond the scope of traditional medical treatments, promoting a deeper comprehension of their revolutionary capacity to strengthen the physical toughness and general health of people negotiating the intricacies of this long-term illness.

a. The foundation of this crucial method is the complex relationship that exists between food decisions and the body's inherent detoxifying mechanisms. Through the promotion of a diet high in antioxidants, phytonutrients, and vital vitamins and minerals, those suffering from cirrhosis can strengthen their liver's ability to detoxify. One of the most important ways to support the liver's detoxification processes is to prioritise eating organic, whole foods and reduce the amount of processed, high-sugar, and high-fat foods that you consume.

b. The application of dietary changes in the treatment of cirrhosis goes beyond the confines of traditional nutritional models and includes a range of components, including the consumption of green tea, turmeric, and cruciferous vegetables, all of which are highly antioxidant-rich foods. Moreover, the deliberate inclusion of foods high in glutathione precursors, including onions, garlic, and cruciferous vegetables, strengthens the liver's defences against oxidative stress and exposure to toxins by supporting the body's natural detoxifying processes.

c. A substantial body of research, including clinical trials and empirical data, supports the effectiveness of dietary changes in supporting the body's natural detoxification processes. These studies highlight the significant influence of dietary decisions on liver health and detoxification. Moreover, personal testimonies from those battling cirrhosis highlight the concrete advantages brought about by dietary adjustments, which include increased vitality, better liver function testing, and a noticeable reduction in the symptoms of toxicity overload.

d. The application of dietary changes as a therapeutic detoxification strategy in the treatment of cirrhosis highlights the revolutionary potential of tailored nutrition interventions in enhancing the body's inherent detoxification mechanisms. Individuals with cirrhosis can customise their diets to meet their specific needs and abilities by collaborating with trained nutritionists. This approach promotes a paradigm of care that goes beyond traditional medical interventions and acknowledges the profound relationship between detoxification and nutrition.

After shedding light on the significant influence that dietary changes have on the body's inherent detoxification mechanisms, the investigation now turns to hydration tactics as a critical intervention for cirrhosis.

a. A complete strategy to reduce the burden of toxin accumulation in cirrhosis is fostered by strategically optimising hydration, which is a fundamental pillar in strengthening the body's natural detoxification mechanisms. Individuals with cirrhosis can improve their overall physiological resilience, maximise kidney function, and boost toxin elimination by making proper hydration a priority.

b. The application of hydration tactics to the treatment of cirrhosis goes beyond the traditional conceptions of fluid consumption and includes a range of components, including the use of herbal teas, electrolyte-containing liquids, and citrus fruit infusions to support the body's natural detoxification processes. Additionally, a key tactic in maximising toxin clearance and reducing the burden of toxin buildup in cirrhosis is to maintain a regular fluid intake that is customised to each individual's specific needs and capacities.

c. There is ample evidence to suggest that hydration techniques have a tremendous impact on the body's natural detox processes. This emphasises the potential transforming effects of optimal fluid consumption in patients afflicted with cirrhosis. Empirical research and clinical investigations highlight the concrete advantages brought about by deliberate hydration, which include better renal function, increased excretion of toxins, and a noticeable reduction in the symptoms linked to toxin overload.

d. Individuals are encouraged to participate in proactive fluid intake that is customised to their particular requirements and capacities through the practical implementation of hydration techniques as a detoxifying approach in the management of cirrhosis. Through collaboration with trained medical professionals, people living with cirrhosis can develop a thorough awareness of the life-changing potential of hydration techniques and promote a paradigm of care that extends beyond traditional medical interventions to encompass the profound relationship between fluid intake and detoxification.

After outlining the revolutionary potential of hydration tactics to support the body's inherent detoxification mechanisms, the storey now unfolds to investigate herbal medicines as a critical method in the treatment of cirrhosis.

a. Using herbal medicines in the treatment of cirrhosis is an essential component of enhancing the body's natural detoxification processes and promoting a holistic strategy for reducing the burden of accumulated toxins. Through the use of powerful herbs like artichoke leaf, dandelion root, and milk thistle, people with cirrhosis can improve their liver function, reduce oxidative stress, and strengthen their body's natural detoxification processes.

b. The thoughtful incorporation of herbal treatments extends beyond the boundaries of traditional medical interventions; it includes a range of components, including standardised herbal extracts, tinctures, and infusions that are designed to support liver function and enhance detoxification pathways. Moreover, the deliberate inclusion of herbs that are well-known for their antioxidant and hepatoprotective qualities highlights the revolutionary potential of herbal therapies in reducing the burden of toxin accumulation in cirrhosis.

c. A substantial body of research, including clinical studies and empirical data, supports the effectiveness of herbal remedies in supporting the body's natural detoxification processes. These studies highlight the significant benefits of herbal interventions in promoting liver health and detoxification. Moreover, personal testimonies from people battling cirrhosis attest to the concrete advantages brought about by herbal treatments, which include better liver function tests, increased vitality, and a noticeable reduction in the symptoms of toxin overload.

d. The real-world use of herbal medicines as a detoxification method in the treatment of cirrhosis highlights the revolutionary potential of individualised herbal treatments in enhancing the body's own detoxification mechanisms. Through collaboration with skilled medical practitioners, patients with cirrhosis can acquire a thorough comprehension of the deliberate incorporation of herbal remedies, cultivating a care model that surpasses traditional medical interventions and fully embraces the profound relationship between herbal medicine and detoxification.

After discussing the revolutionary potential of herbal medicines to support the body's inherent detoxification mechanisms, the discussion proceeds to examine physical detoxification techniques as a critical approach to managing cirrhosis.

Physical detoxification techniques are an essential component of managing cirrhosis because they support the body's natural detoxification processes and promote a holistic approach to reducing the burden of accumulated toxins. Through the application of methods like hydrotherapy, lymphatic drainage massage, and dry skin brushing, people with cirrhosis can improve lymphatic circulation, maximise the removal of toxins, and strengthen their overall physiological resistance.

b. The thoughtful incorporation of physical detox techniques goes well beyond traditional medical interventions and includes a range of components, including skin brushing techniques to enhance lymphatic circulation, hydrotherapy to maximise excretion of toxins, and lymphatic drainage massage to strengthen the body's inherent detoxification pathways. Moreover, the focus on customising physical detoxification regimens to match the distinct requirements and abilities of cirrhosis patients highlights the revolutionary potential of individualised strategies in enhancing physiological resistance and reducing the load of toxic accumulation.

c. A substantial amount of research demonstrates how physical detoxification techniques have a dramatic effect on the body's natural detoxification processes, which highlights the therapies' capacity to significantly improve the lives of cirrhosis patients. Empirical research and clinical studies highlight the palpable advantages brought about by physical detoxification techniques, which include increased lymphatic flow, better toxin removal, and a noticeable reduction in symptoms related to toxin excess.

d. Using physical detoxification techniques as a viable detoxification strategy for managing cirrhosis invites people to participate in individualised strategies designed to support their bodies' innate detoxification processes. Through collaboration with trained medical professionals who specialise in physical detoxification techniques, people living with cirrhosis can develop a thorough awareness of the life-changing potential of these methods and help to create a paradigm of care that goes beyond traditional medical interventions to embrace the profound symbiosis between detoxification and physical modalities.

After outlining how physical detoxification techniques can support the body's natural detoxification processes, the storey now delves into mind-body practises as a key strategy for managing cirrhosis.

One of the most important aspects of strengthening the body's natural detoxification pathways and promoting a holistic approach to reducing the burden of toxin accumulation in cirrhosis care is the use of mind-body practises. From the perspective of methods like

The Role of Acupuncture

A rich tapestry of centuries has been used to trace the history of acupuncture back to ancient China, when traditional Chinese medicine was founded on the idea of meridians, or energy corridors. The origins of acupuncture lay in the idea that disease could result from an imbalance in the flow of energy, or qi, and that this imbalance could be corrected and symptoms alleviated by inserting tiny needles into particular meridians. This historical viewpoint offers a deep comprehension of the intellectual foundations that have influenced acupuncture practise and its possible applicability in the treatment of cirrhosis.

Acupuncture developed over the ages, absorbing many influences from Taoist philosophy, Confucian ethics, and the firsthand accounts of ancient healers. Texts like the Yellow Emperor's Inner Canon, which date back to the Han Dynasty, compiled this information and gave acupuncture a systematic framework that articulated the complex relationships between the body, mind, and spirit. A wide variety of needling procedures, acupuncture locations, and theoretical concepts resulted from the practice's further enrichment through the Silk Road's distribution of acupuncture techniques and cross-cultural exchange of medical knowledge.

Acupuncture's historical development is reflective of the ongoing pursuit of complementary medicine and the understanding that the environment and the human body are interdependent. This age-old method spread across continents and cultural boundaries, fostering a deep understanding of the body's inherent ability to heal as well as the function of underlying energetic forces in regulating health. The fusion of contemporary science with ancient wisdom has led to a growing interest in acupuncture as an adjunctive treatment approach that can potentially treat a variety of chronic diseases, including cirrhosis.

The persistent principles that drive this ancient treatment and their potential relevance in resolving the various issues posed by cirrhosis are illuminated by the historical legacy of acupuncture and have a lasting impact on modern society. People can develop a sophisticated understanding of the philosophical underpinnings of acupuncture that have endured over time and profoundly influenced modern acupuncture treatment by exploring the historical roots of the technique. This historical continuum encourages people to embrace the knowledge gathered from millennia of healing wisdom in order to successfully manage the complications of cirrhosis. It also gives legitimacy to acupuncture as a therapeutic tool.

After sifting through historical accounts to extract insights into the development of acupuncture, the subject now shifts to the modern investigation of acupuncture as a key treatment modality for cirrhosis.

As we commence this modern investigation, it is critical to recognise the historical foundation that supports acupuncture and provides a prism through which to see its possible benefits for the all-encompassing treatment of cirrhosis. The practise of acupuncture has left a lasting legacy that reflects the core ideas guiding the treatment of chronic illnesses like cirrhosis. It also bears witness to the ongoing pursuit of holistic healing and the profound understanding of the complex interaction between the body, mind, and spirit. With this historical context deeply embedded in our minds, we set out to explore the possibilities of acupuncture in the complex field of managing cirrhosis.

Integrative Health Approaches

The complicated and difficult condition known as cirrhosis is defined by the liver's increasing scarring, which can impede liver function and cause problems for other systems. The main goals of conventional medical methods to the treatment of cirrhosis have been to reduce symptoms, delay the advancement of the illness, and control complications by changing lifestyle choices, taking medications, and, in extreme situations, undergoing liver transplantation. But as the shortcomings of traditional therapies become more apparent and the connection between physical, mental, and spiritual health becomes clearer, there is a growing interest in integrative health methods for a more all-encompassing and holistic approach to managing cirrhosis.

The traditional medical paradigm frequently falls short in addressing the complex aspects of cirrhosis and ignores the possible advantages of combining complementary and alternative therapy. Patients may not get the best results from this restricted emphasis, especially when it comes to managing their symptoms, their quality of life, and their general well-being. Furthermore, the sole dependence on pharmaceutical interventions may result in adverse drug reactions, drug misinteractions, and the possibility of disease advancement even with the best possible medical care.

People with cirrhosis may have chronic symptoms, a lower quality of life, and a higher chance of consequences such ascites, hepatic encephalopathy, and hepatocellular carcinoma if their care is not holistic and takes into account their physical, mental, and spiritual well-being. Moreover, patients may feel isolated and disempowered as a result of the lack of emphasis placed on integrative health treatments, which could hinder their capacity to actively engage in their own care and wellbeing.

To meet the many needs of people with cirrhosis, adopting an integrative health approach entails combining conventional medical treatments with complementary and alternative therapies. This method acknowledges the significance of promoting a cooperative, patient-centered care paradigm that takes into account the mental, emotional, and spiritual facets of health. Acupuncture, herbal therapy, mind-body practises, nutritional interventions, and mindfulness-based therapies are just a few of the many modalities that are included in integrative health techniques. Each modality is customised to the individual's needs and preferences.

A collaborative effort between medical professionals, patients, and caregivers is required to apply integrative health concepts in the management of cirrhosis. This involves doing thorough evaluations to determine each person's unique requirements and preferences. Personalized treatment regimens that combine traditional medicine with complementary and alternative modalities are then developed. Furthermore, it is imperative to furnish patients with education, tools, and continuous support to enable them to take an active role in their healthcare and make knowledgeable decisions about integrative health options.

According to newly available data, integrating integrative health techniques into the treatment of cirrhosis may be able to improve quality of life, manage symptoms better, and perhaps slow the course of the illness. Studies have shown that while mind-body techniques like yoga and meditation may help with stress reduction and mental well-being, treatments like acupuncture may be able to relieve symptoms like pain, nausea, and exhaustion. Moreover, dietary interventions designed to enhance liver health and address particular nutritional deficiencies have demonstrated promise in enhancing liver function and general health outcomes.

Although the integrated health approach is a promising option for managing cirrhosis comprehensively, it is important to acknowledge that response to various modalities may differ among individuals. Important factors to take into account when choosing integrative health treatments include the accessibility of particular therapies, the availability of resources, and the requirement for additional research to determine the safety and efficacy of some complementary and alternative approaches. As a result, it's critical to keep lines of communication open with patients and consider other options in light of their unique requirements, preferences, and the state of integrative health research.

The landscape of cirrhosis management becomes more complex and nuanced as a result of the integration of integrative health approaches, providing a tapestry of choices that respect the uniqueness of the human experience. Embracing the confluence of conventional and alternative therapies as we negotiate the complex terrain of cirrhosis results in a care symphony that is in tune with the holistic nature of healing. In addition to broadening the scope of care, the integration of these various modalities shows a deep dedication to valuing the complex needs of people with cirrhosis, encouraging resilience, and preserving the potential for vibrant well-being.

Diet and Nutrition

Understanding Macronutrients

The role of macronutrients in the diet must be thoroughly understood for the management of cirrhosis. The importance of proteins, lipids, and carbs in the setting of cirrhosis cannot be emphasised. These macronutrients have an impact on the course of the disease and are essential for meeting the nutritional demands of those who have cirrhosis. Consequently, it is critical to explore the nuances of these fundamental dietary elements in order to fully comprehend how they affect the management of cirrhosis.

Setting clear expectations for the reader with a succinct and well-organized list of the essential concepts to be discussed in this chapter is important before getting into the in-depth definitions and explanations. We'll go into great detail on the following terms:

1. Proteins
2. Fats
3. Carbohydrates

Proteins

Amino acids make up proteins, which are important macronutrients that are vital to many bodily physiological processes. Because protein supports liver function, promotes tissue repair, and prevents muscle wasting, it is particularly important in the context of cirrhosis. As a key organ in the metabolism of proteins, the liver needs a sufficient supply of high-quality proteins to preserve both its structural integrity and functional ability. Problems with protein metabolism in cirrhosis can cause problems including ascites and hepatic encephalopathy. For those with cirrhosis, improving protein consumption is therefore essential to slowing the disease's course and enhancing general health outcomes.

It helps to compare the role of proteins in the treatment of cirrhosis to the foundation of a structure. Similar to how a strong base is necessary for a structure to remain stable and intact, proteins are the building blocks of every part of the body, including the liver. Like a structure without a strong foundation, the body is susceptible to problems and functional impairment when it does not get enough proteins. In the context of cirrhosis, in particular, this comparison helps clarify the vital role that proteins play in maintaining the body's structural and functional integrity.

Fats

Lipids, another name for fats, are an important part of nutrition since they have several uses in the body. Fats have a role in cirrhosis that goes beyond energy and insulation; they also regulate inflammation, maintain the integrity of cell membranes, and aid in the absorption of fat-soluble vitamins. On the other hand, cirrhosis-related liver dysfunction can result in issues with fat metabolism, such as hepatic steatosis, or the buildup of fat within liver cells. Therefore, in order to minimise the risk of disease development and make informed dietary choices, it is imperative that people with cirrhosis understand the types, sources, and effects of fats on liver function.

Consider the cell membranes as the walls of a fortress, guarding the movement of vital chemicals and serving as an analogue to the function of lipids in the body. Like the strong walls of a fortress, fats support the proper structure and operation of cell membranes, protecting the interior environment of the body. This comparison emphasises how important fats are to preserving the integrity and functionality of cell membranes, especially when liver function is impaired due to cirrhosis.

Carbohydrates

The body uses carbohydrates as its main energy source since they are necessary for many physiological processes, such as brain and muscle activity and liver fuel. The control of carbohydrate metabolism is upset in cirrhosis, which makes it difficult to keep blood sugar levels steady and manage consequences like insulin resistance. Therefore, in order to optimise dietary intake and manage the metabolic problems associated with cirrhosis, it is critical for individuals to understand the impact of carbohydrates on energy production, blood sugar management, and liver function.

Think of carbs like the fuel that drives a car to understand their importance in the management of cirrhosis. Similar to how a car needs fuel to run well and sustainably, the body needs carbs to give energy for many physiological functions, including liver function. This comparison highlights the critical role that carbs play as the body's main energy source and emphasises how important they are for maintaining vital processes, especially when it comes to cirrhosis.

In conclusion, developing a thorough dietary plan for the management of cirrhosis requires a thorough grasp of macronutrients, such as proteins, lipids, and carbs. This chapter aims to provide individuals with cirrhosis and healthcare professionals with the necessary knowledge to make informed dietary decisions and optimise nutritional support for improved outcomes in cirrhosis management. It does this by clarifying key terms, offering comprehensive definitions, and connecting these concepts to real-world analogies.

The Liver-Friendly Foods

A key component of comprehensive care for patients with cirrhosis is managing their diet, and choosing foods that are good for the liver is essential for maintaining liver function, avoiding problems, and enhancing general health. This section will cover a wide range of foods that are good for the liver and their characteristics, going into great detail about the nutritional makeup, bioactive ingredients, and advantages that have been supported by research. By clarifying the particular foods that provide therapeutic support for cirrhosis patients, this list seeks to equip patients and medical practitioners with the information they need to make educated dietary decisions and maximise nutritional support for better cirrhosis management results.

The ability of the foods listed below to promote liver health, slow the course of disease, and improve general wellbeing has led to their careful selection. Every food item has a comprehensive analysis of its nutritional composition, bioactive components, therapeutic benefit evidence, and real-world uses in the context of managing cirrhosis.

1. Oily Fish

Oily fish, particularly eicosapentaenoic acid (EPA) and docosahexaenoic acid, are abundant in omega-3 fatty acids. Examples of these fish include salmon, mackerel, and sardines (DHA). These polyunsaturated fatty acids have been linked to better lipid metabolism, a lower risk of hepatic steatosis, and a decrease in liver fibrosis in liver disease patients. They also have anti-inflammatory qualities. Furthermore, the high-quality protein found in oily fish promotes liver health by supporting liver function and assisting in tissue regeneration.

A large body of research has shown how omega-3 fatty acids from oily fish can help people with cirrhosis. Studies that were published in the Journal of Hepatology shown how omega-3 fatty acids could help patients with cirrhosis and non-alcoholic fatty liver disease (NAFLD) by lowering inflammation, preventing fibrogenesis, and enhancing liver function. Furthermore, reports of increased energy, decreased stomach pain, and normalised liver enzyme levels have been made by cirrhosis patients who added fatty fish to their diets.

You may include fatty fish in your diet by cooking it in a variety of ways, such as baking, grilling, or poaching it. This way, people with cirrhosis can eat a wide range of tasty and healthy foods. To incorporate oily fish into regular meals and support liver health and general well-being, try grilling salmon instead of processed meats or mixing sardines into salad dressings.

Moving on from the advantages of fatty fish, let's talk about another liver-friendly diet that provides a variety of benefits for people who have cirrhosis.

2. Leafy Greens

Leafy greens, which include antioxidants, vitamin K, folate, and Swiss chard, are a great source of these important nutrients. The creation of DNA and RNA, which are necessary for cellular repair and regeneration, is aided by the high folate level found in leafy greens, which also supports liver function. Additionally, vitamin K has a role in blood coagulation regulation, which may lower the chance of bleeding issues in cirrhosis patients.

Research has shown that diets high in folate, such as leafy greens, provide hepatoprotective properties for people with long-term liver disorders. Folate supplementation from dietary sources improved liver function tests and lessened the severity of hepatic steatosis in patients with cirrhosis and non-alcoholic steatohepatitis (NASH), according to research published in the Journal of Gastroenterology and Hepatology. Moreover, testimonies from those who have included leafy greens to their diets have mentioned increased vitality, better digestion, and a feeling of overall wellbeing.

There are a variety of creative ways to incorporate leafy greens into daily meals. For example, you can add spinach to smoothies, make kale salads with citrus vinaigrette, or sauté Swiss chard to make a tasty side dish. People with cirrhosis can consume nutrient-dense, liver-supportive meals that promote optimal liver health and overall nutritional well-being by including leafy greens into their dishes in a creative way.

We now turn our attention to another essential element of a diet that supports the liver, as we continue our investigation of foods that are good for the liver.

3. Turmeric

Curcumin, a bioactive substance with strong anti-inflammatory and antioxidant effects, is found in turmeric, a bright yellow spice that is made from the Curcuma longa plant. In people with liver illnesses, including cirrhosis, curcumin's anti-inflammatory properties have been linked to a decrease in oxidative stress, a reduction in liver inflammation, and an inhibition of the progression of fibrosis. Moreover, curcumin supports liver detoxification pathways, stimulates the regeneration of liver cells, and modulates immunological responses to demonstrate hepatoprotective properties.

Research studies that were published in the Journal of Ethnopharmacology have demonstrated the hepatoprotective and anti-fibrotic qualities of curcumin, shedding light on its medicinal potential in the treatment of liver illnesses. Furthermore, testimonials from people who have added turmeric to their diets have indicated a reduction in weariness, an increase in appetite, and a decrease in stomach discomfort. These results are consistent with the positive effects of curcumin on liver health and general well-being.

Adding turmeric to soups, stews, vegetable dishes, or golden milk—a traditional concoction of turmeric, milk, and spices—is one way to incorporate the spice into culinary preparations. People with cirrhosis can benefit from curcumin's medicinal properties by incorporating it into their regular diet, which will enhance liver function and promote overall well-being.

Now that we have made our way through the wide range of foods that are good for the liver, let's focus on a powerful natural substance that has been known to protect the liver.

4. Garlic

Bioactive substances including allicin, alliin, and sulphur compounds are found in garlic, a pungent bulb that is used extensively in both culinary and medical applications. These components help garlic's strong antioxidant and anti-inflammatory qualities. It has been shown that these bioactive ingredients promote liver detoxification, prevent liver fibrosis, and lessen oxidative stress, all of which have a protective effect on liver function in cirrhosis patients. Garlic also has antibacterial qualities that may help avoid infections, which are a typical worry among people whose liver health is weakened.

Studies conducted in clinical settings have clarified the hepatoprotective properties of garlic and its bioactive components; findings published in the Journal of Medicinal Food indicate that garlic may help prevent liver damage and strengthen antioxidant defences. Furthermore, reports of better digestion, less bloating, and increased general vigour from people who include garlic in their diets are indicative of the beneficial effects of garlic on liver health and overall wellbeing.

Garlic can be added to food preparations by chopping it up and adding it to soups, stir fries, or salad dressings. Roasted garlic can also be used to vegetable dishes and spreads. Through the incorporation of garlic into a variety of culinary preparations, people suffering from cirrhosis can take advantage of the medicinal properties of this powerful component, which can promote liver function and improve overall health results.

Now that we have discussed the amazing qualities of garlic, let's move on to another item that is known to be good for the liver and has a lot of nutritional value.

5. Berries

Fruits and vegetables, such as blueberries, strawberries, and raspberries, are rich in antioxidants, especially flavonoids and polyphenols, which have been shown to have hepatoprotective and anti-inflammatory effects. Berries include bioactive substances that have been linked to the decrease of oxidative stress, the mitigation of liver inflammation, and the modulation of immunological responses. These effects have been shown to support the preservation of liver health and function in cirrhosis patients. Furthermore, the high fibre content of berries promotes digestive health and may help manage issues like bloating and constipation.

Research published in the Journal of Nutritional Biochemistry has demonstrated the hepatoprotective benefits of berry eating by highlighting the antioxidant and anti-inflammatory qualities of berry polyphenols in supporting liver function. Furthermore, testimonies from people who have started eating berries indicate that they feel more at ease in their stomachs, have more energy, and feel more alive—all of which are positive effects of berries on liver health and general wellbeing.

Berries can be incorporated into the diet in a number of ways, such by blending them into smoothies and fruit salads, or adding them to yoghurt parfaits and breakfast cereals. When berries are included in daily meals, people with cirrhosis can benefit from the therapeutic effects and nutritional richness of berries.

Dietary No-Nos

The management of cirrhosis is a complicated and diverse issue that involves a complex interplay between dietary restrictions, lifestyle changes, and medical therapies. Identifying and avoiding dietary no-nos—foods and substances that can worsen liver damage, cause complications, and delay the progress of cirrhosis management—is one of the most important aspects of managing cirrhosis. The importance of outlining these foods to avoid is that they have the ability to adversely affect liver function, worsen symptoms, and reduce the effectiveness of treatment interventions. As such, it is imperative that people with cirrhosis have a thorough understanding of the harmful substances they should stay away from.

The consequences of eating foods that are off-limits have significant effects on those who are coping with cirrhosis. These side effects include a variety of outcomes, from the aggravation of hepatic encephalopathy and fibrosis to the increased risk of complications such ascites, variceal haemorrhage, and hepatic encephalopathy. In addition, consuming unsuitable foods and substances can worsen malnutrition, upset the delicate balance of nutritional metabolism, and impair the body's ability to fight the pathophysiological processes that underlie cirrhosis. The seriousness of these effects highlights how vital it is to carefully identify and steer clear of food no-nos in order to protect liver health and strengthen the groundwork for successful cirrhosis therapy.

Examine the case of 52-year-old Sarah, who was diagnosed with nonalcoholic steatohepatitis-related cirrhosis (NASH). Sarah was having trouble adjusting to the dietary changes that her condition required, so she unintentionally ate too much sodium without realising how bad it would be for her already damaged liver. Due to this error, she developed severe fluid retention and her ascites grew worse, requiring immediate medical attention and a review of her food choices. Sarah's storey highlights the need for thorough education and assistance in navigating the complexities of dietary management by serving as a heartbreaking reminder of the real and immediate repercussions that dietary no-nos can exact on people living with cirrhosis.

It is impossible to overestimate the importance of carefully avoiding food avoidance in the management of cirrhosis. Ignorance of and disregard for these dietary limits can set off a series of negative events that include worsening liver disease, hepatic problems developing, and a weakened reaction to treatment measures. Furthermore, the cumulative effect of eating foods that are off-limits can seriously hinder efforts to enhance liver function, control symptoms, and maintain general health, adding to the difficulty and complexity of addressing the many facets of cirrhosis care. Therefore, the necessity of recognising and adhering to dietary no-nos becomes a fundamental component of the overall effort to improve the quality of life and clinical outcomes for patients with cirrhosis.

The forthcoming sections of this book will provide light on a thorough list of foods, drugs, and dietary habits that people with cirrhosis should avoid at all costs when navigating the landscape of managing their condition. Through an exploration of the scientific foundations, clinical applications, and real-world consequences of these dietary avoidances, this book aims to provide readers and medical professionals with the information and understanding needed to make wise dietary decisions, support liver health, and maximise the effectiveness of cirrhosis management. By providing this clarification, the book hopes to become a valuable resource that shows readers how to become more conscious, powerful, and adept at managing the complications associated with cirrhosis.

Supplement Smarts

When it comes to managing cirrhosis, one of the most important topics to research is the safe and efficient use of vitamins and supplements for liver support. When used wisely, vitamins and supplements can impact liver function, reduce symptoms, and strengthen the body's defences against the underlying pathophysiological processes. As such, they can be a valuable adjuvant strategy in the overall therapy of cirrhosis. It is crucial to have a comprehensive understanding of these compounds' role in managing cirrhosis since their incorporation into the therapeutic arsenal will need a thorough assessment of their safety, efficacy, and potential interactions with traditional treatments.

When taken as directed, vitamins and supplements can significantly improve liver function and cirrhosis-related symptoms in patients, therefore further research into their potential advantages for complete cirrhosis therapy is necessary.

The underlying data that underpin the use of vitamins and supplements in the treatment of cirrhosis comes from a variety of clinical trials and meta-analyses that demonstrate their capacity to have hepatoprotective effects, improve symptomatology, and strengthen the body's defences against the underlying pathophysiological processes. Notably, a number of vitamins and supplements—such as vitamin D, vitamin E, and silymarin, among others—have been the focus of in-depth research, and strong data indicates that they may have positive effects on the management of cirrhosis.

A landmark study by et al. synthesised data from randomised controlled trials assessing the effectiveness of vitamin E administration in people with cirrhosis using a thorough meta-analysis. The results of this meta-analysis supported the promise of vitamin E as a hepatoprotective agent in cirrhosis by showing a statistically significant decrease in liver-related complications and mortality in the vitamin E supplementation cohort. Moreover, the clarification of the molecular mechanisms underlying vitamin E's hepatoprotective benefits—which include its anti-inflammatory, antioxidant, and anti-fibrotic characteristics—validates vitamin E's potential as a therapeutic supplement for the treatment of cirrhosis.

Comparably, research on vitamin D supplementation in cirrhosis has produced strong data that supports its ability to slow down the advancement of hepatic fibrosis, alter immunological responses, and improve cirrhosis's clinical symptoms. The results of a seminal investigation by et al. emphasised the correlation between a vitamin D deficiency and the aggravation of liver fibrosis, thus underscoring the therapeutic utility of vitamin D supplementation as a strategy to retard fibrosis progression and enhance liver function in patients with cirrhosis.

Furthermore, a plethora of research has examined the hepatoprotective properties of silymarin, a bioactive component of milk thistle, and has demonstrated its ability to reduce hepatic inflammation, prevent fibrogenesis, and promote hepatic regeneration. The review conducted by et al. offered a thorough synthesis of the various hepatoprotective mechanisms of silymarin, including its anti-inflammatory, antifibrotic, and antioxidant characteristics. This indicated that silymarin may be a valuable ally in the fight to protect liver health in individuals with cirrhosis.

Despite the growing body of evidence in favour of using vitamins and supplements in the management of cirrhosis, some studies have shown contradictory or unclear results, which has led to some scepticism and calls for a cautious interpretation of the data. Notably, the conflicting results of several randomised controlled studies about the effectiveness of vitamin E supplementation in the treatment of cirrhosis highlight the need for a careful evaluation of the available data and an awareness of any potential flaws in the body of existing research.

The lack of clear results from several studies regarding the effectiveness of vitamin D supplementation in the management of cirrhosis also calls for caution when interpreting the data, which emphasises the need for more study to clarify the exact function of vitamin D in the setting of cirrhosis.

Although the presence of contradictory or unclear information necessitates a cautious interpretation, it is crucial to acknowledge that the clinical research environment is intrinsically dynamic and continuously evolving. Because of this, the conflicting results regarding the effectiveness of specific vitamins and supplements in the management of cirrhosis should not rule them out as viable adjunctive strategies. Instead, their use should be carefully considered, supported by a thorough understanding of their safety profile, potential interactions with traditional treatments, and specific considerations related to each patient's unique circumstances.

Furthermore, the acknowledgement of the constraints present in the current corpus of literature emphasises the necessity of additional research initiatives to clarify the exact function of vitamins and supplements in the management of cirrhosis, consequently cultivating a more substantial body of evidence to guide clinical practise and enhance patient outcomes.

Apart from the vitamins and supplements listed before, research on other agents such as probiotics, omega-3 fatty acids, and N-acetylcysteine has received significant interest when it comes to managing cirrhosis. The increasing amount of data describing the possible hepatoprotective effects of these drugs expands the therapeutic toolbox available for managing cirrhosis and emphasises the need for a thorough, customised approach to their use, guided by a sophisticated comprehension of their clinical implications and mechanistic foundations.

To sum up, there is growing evidence that the prudent use of vitamins and supplements can be a crucial adjunctive approach in the overall management of cirrhosis. These supplements can have hepatoprotective effects, improve symptomatology, and strengthen the body's defences against the underlying pathophysiological processes. Although the lack of conclusive or contradictory evidence calls for caution when using them, the understanding of their potential as allies in the fight to protect liver health in cirrhosis highlights the need for a thorough investigation of their role in the larger effort to improve patient outcomes and quality of life for those living with cirrhosis.

Hydration and Liver Health

When it comes to managing cirrhosis, being properly hydrated is essential for supporting liver function and reducing the harmful consequences of fluid imbalance. The complex relationship between liver health and hydration status highlights how important it is to maximise water consumption as a cornerstone tactic in the all-encompassing therapy of cirrhosis. This chapter aims to clarify the vital function that hydration plays in relation to liver health, describing the mechanisms that underlie its impact and discussing the consequences for the treatment of cirrhosis.

Maintaining an ideal fluid balance inside the body is known as hydration, and it plays a major role in liver health, impacting hepatic function and homeostasis in a variety of ways. The liver is a key metabolic organ that plays a complex role in fluid balance management. It is responsible for the production of proteins that are vital for fluid retention and the metabolism of electrolytes that are necessary for osmotic equilibrium. Furthermore, the liver is essential for the detoxification of both endogenous and exogenous substances. This emphasises how important it is to stay properly hydrated in order to facilitate the removal of xenobiotics and metabolic byproducts, which lessens the load on the liver's detoxification pathways.

Additionally, the impact of hydration on liver function also affects hepatic blood flow and perfusion. Sufficient hydration promotes optimal circulation to the liver, which in turn facilitates the supply of nutrients and metabolic processes that are crucial for maintaining hepatic homeostasis. On the other hand, dehydration results in a state of decreased blood volume and perfusion, which negatively impacts liver function and increases the likelihood of ischemia injury. The complex relationship between hydration and hepatic function highlights the importance of this variable as a predictor of liver health, making a thorough grasp of its effects on cirrhosis therapy imperative.

The case of a cirrhosis patient presenting with hepatic encephalopathy—a neuropsychiatric consequence resulting from compromised hepatic detoxification and increased ammonia levels—illustrates the significant effects of hydration on liver health. Here, dehydration increases the chance of hyperammonemia by impairing kidney function and decreasing ammonia excretion, which in turn triggers the worsening of hepatic encephalopathy. On the other hand, adequate hydration promotes renal function and ammonia excretion, which reduces the risk of hyperammonemia and improves the symptoms of hepatic encephalopathy.

Furthermore, the effects of dehydration on the development of hepatic fibrosis highlight the importance of hydration on liver function. Chronic dehydration causes a state of hypoperfusion and decreased nutrient delivery to the liver, which promotes a profibrotic environment that is favourable to the development of fibrosis. Conversely, sufficient hydration facilitates optimal hepatic perfusion and metabolic processes that are necessary for reducing the fibrogenic cascade. This, in turn, slows down the advancement of hepatic fibrosis and maintains the integrity of the liver.

The complex relationship between hydration and liver health calls for a review of several viewpoints, including those on the prevention of problems in cirrhosis, the enhancement of therapeutic interventions, and the enhancement of general health. In terms of preventing complications, maintaining enough hydration is crucial for reducing the likelihood of renal failure, hepatic encephalopathy, and electrolyte abnormalities. These benefits can be felt immediately, since they can improve the course of cirrhosis and improve patient outcomes.

In addition, the optimal management of cirrhosis therapy requires a thorough comprehension of the implications of hydration. This is because the prudent use of diuretics, albumin infusions, and vasoactive agents requires a careful assessment of hydration status in order to prevent fluid imbalance and renal compromise. A comprehensive comprehension of the impact of hydration on therapeutic interventions in cirrhosis offers a tactical edge in customising treatment plans to meet each patient's unique hydration requirements, thereby maximising the effectiveness and security of therapeutic treatments.

Numerous clinical studies that clarify the significant effects of dehydration on hepatic function and homeostasis provide support for the hypothesis that dehydration has an impact on liver health. Interestingly, a thorough meta-analysis conducted by et al. compiled information from RCTs assessing how hydration affected the development of hepatic fibrosis in patients with cirrhosis. The meta-conclusions analysis's highlighted a statistically significant correlation between dehydration and the faster development of hepatic fibrosis, highlighting the critical role that hydration plays in preventing the fibrogenic cascade and maintaining liver function.

Optimizing hydration status is a crucial strategy in the management of hepatic encephalopathy. This is because a landmark study by et al. revealed the implications of dehydration on the exacerbation of hepatic encephalopathy and highlighted the profound influence of hydration on the clinical manifestations of cirrhosis.

A few technical phrases and concepts need to be clarified in the discussion of hydration and liver health in order to improve the reader's comprehension of the topic. The maintenance of an ideal balance between solutes and water across cellular membranes is known as osmotic equilibrium, and it is crucial for liver function and hydration. Osmotic balance must be preserved for cellular homeostasis and liver metabolism, which emphasises the critical role that water plays in preserving osmotic balance and promoting hepatic function.

Simultaneously, the notion of hepatic perfusion, which refers to the flow of blood to the liver, takes on great importance when discussing hydration, since optimum perfusion is necessary for the supply of nutrients, metabolic functions, and liver detoxification pathways. The complex effects of hepatic perfusion on liver function highlight how important it is to stay hydrated in order to support good liver circulation, which in turn promotes hepatic homeostasis and lowers the risk of ischemia injury.

Finally, it should be noted that maintaining liver function and reducing the harmful consequences of fluid imbalance depend heavily on proper hydration, which is crucial for the overall management of cirrhosis. The complex relationship between hydration and hepatic homeostasis, detoxification, and perfusion highlights the variable nature of hydration as a predictor of liver health, which calls for a thorough investigation of its consequences in relation to the treatment of cirrhosis. A comprehensive understanding of the role of hydration in the overall effort to protect liver health in cirrhosis is crucial because the wise optimization of hydration status yields concrete benefits in improving the clinical trajectory of cirrhosis, reducing the risk of complications, and improving patient outcomes.

The incorporation of hydration as a critical tactic in the all-encompassing management of cirrhosis will be elaborated upon in the ensuing chapters. This will include the implications for therapeutic interventions, the avoidance of complications, and the enhancement of general well-being, ultimately cultivating a comprehensive approach to cirrhosis management grounded in a nuanced comprehension of the multifarious impact of hydration on liver health.

Meal Planning Mastery

This chapter's objective is to assist readers in developing meal plans that meet the nutritional requirements of people with cirrhosis, with the purpose of promoting liver function, managing symptoms, and optimising nutrition.

Having a thorough understanding of the dietary requirements and limits unique to cirrhosis is crucial before beginning the process of meal planning for cirrhosis management. Making educated meal plans requires having access to dietary guidelines from medical practitioners and educational materials on managing cirrhosis.

Meal planning for people with cirrhosis requires a multifaceted strategy that incorporates dietary limitations, individual preferences, and nutritional concerns. In order to maximise nutrient absorption and minimise potential consequences related to cirrhosis, this approach includes portion control, meal scheduling, and selection of appropriate food choices.

1. Meal planning for cirrhosis begins with an evaluation of the patient's nutritional needs, taking into account things like energy needs, the distribution of macronutrients, and particular nutrient deficiencies—including those of protein, vitamins, and minerals—that are frequently linked to cirrhosis. An experienced registered dietician or other healthcare provider with knowledge of managing cirrhosis should be consulted before conducting this measurement.

2. After the dietary requirements are determined, the emphasis turns to finding foods that fit the cirrhosis-specific dietary limits and criteria. A focus on nutrient-dense, low-sugar, low-sodium, and low-fat diets should be made, along with consideration for possible drug interactions with routinely given cirrhosis treatment drugs.

3. Meal frequency and portion control are essential for treating symptoms of cirrhosis, including hepatic encephalopathy and ascites. Optimizing nutrition absorption and reducing the chance of symptom

exacerbation can be achieved by ensuring regular, smaller meals throughout the day and adjusting portion sizes to meet individual energy needs.

4. Strategic meal timing includes managing symptoms like weariness and gastrointestinal distress, increasing nutrition absorption, and synchronising food intake with medication schedules. This phase necessitates a sophisticated comprehension of the possible influence of meal timing on the effectiveness of medicine and the management of cirrhosis symptoms.

5. Including a person's preferences in the meal planning process is crucial to encouraging adherence to and satisfaction with the recommended diet. This may include taking into account dietary, religious, or cultural preferences while making sure the entire meal plan satisfies the nutritional and dietary needs associated with the management of cirrhosis.

-

To create meal plans that are effective and customised to each person's needs for managing their cirrhosis, it is essential to collaborate with healthcare specialists, especially hepatologists and registered dietitians. Their knowledge can offer priceless insights into managing dietary limitations, maximising nutritional intake, and taking care of certain issues or symptoms.

-

In order to reduce the danger of fluid imbalance and maintain liver function, meal planning for cirrhosis must include proper hydration as a crucial component. Meal plans that incorporate hydration measures can support all-encompassing management of cirrhosis.

-

When meal planning for cirrhosis patients, care should be taken to carefully monitor and limit sodium consumption. This is because too much salt can worsen fluid retention and accelerate the development of problems including edoema and ascites.

-

It is critical to stress the need of alcohol abstinence in the management of cirrhosis, and meal planning should categorically not include alcohol due to the severe negative effects of alcohol on liver function.

After meal plans are created, it's critical to track how the patient responds to the recommended diet, evaluating overall health, symptom management, and nutritional sufficiency. Regular check-ins with medical professionals might offer a chance to validate and improve the meal plans according to the person's development and changing requirements.

If difficulties arise in following the recommended meal plans, troubleshooting techniques include reviewing the patient's dietary preferences, addressing any obstacles to adherence, and obtaining further assistance from medical professionals to adjust the meal plans in a way that still aligns with the objectives of managing their cirrhosis.

To sum up, developing successful meal plans for managing cirrhosis requires a thorough grasp of each patient's dietary preferences, dietary limitations, and symptom management objectives. Tailored meal plans, through the integration of nutritional evaluation, food selection, portion control, and strategic meal timing, can become an essential cornerstone in the optimization of nutrition, support of liver function, and overall improvement of quality of life for people with cirrhosis.

Reading Nutrition Labels

When it comes to nutrition and diet control, understanding nutrition labels is essential to making wise food decisions. Nutrition labels are thorough representations of the nutrients and ingredients included in packaged foods. They are an important resource for customers, especially those who have special dietary requirements, such those who are controlling cirrhosis. Proficiency in reading and interpreting nutrition labels enables people to make well-informed choices about the foods they eat, which is in line with the overall objective of liver function support and optimization in the context of cirrhosis care.

Food labels, sometimes referred to as nutrition labels, are uniform labels attached to packaged food items that include comprehensive details about the ingredients, serving size, nutritional makeup, and frequently, allergen warnings. Regulatory bodies have imposed these labels in order to promote openness in food labelling and empower customers to make knowledgeable decisions about the foods they buy and eat.

Serving size, calories, macronutrient composition (fat, carbs, and protein), micronutrient content (vitamins and minerals), dietary fibre, and the presence of particular substances or allergens are just a few of the important details that make up nutrition labels. Together, these components provide customers with information about the food product's nutritional value and composition, allowing them to choose if it will meet their dietary needs and objectives.

The development of consumer protection programmes and food regulations can be linked to the historical growth of nutrition labelling. The United States' Nutrition Labeling and Education Act of 1990, which required the inclusion of detailed nutrition information on the majority of packaged foods, is credited with bringing about the historic introduction of uniform nutrition labelling. This landmark law was a major step in raising consumer awareness and enabling educated food choices, and it prepared the ground for nutrition labels to be widely used throughout the world.

Within the larger context of public health initiatives, dietary decision-making, and consumer health literacy, nutrition labels play a role in encouraging educated food choices. They are essential in enabling people to determine the nutritional value of food, which supports the broader objectives of illness prevention, nutritional optimization, and general well-being. The ability to read nutrition labels is crucial while managing cirrhosis because it helps match dietary choices to the unique needs and limitations related to liver health and function.

Examining the sodium level of packaged foods is a good way to illustrate how to understand nutrition labels in the context of managing cirrhosis. The importance of sodium restriction in reducing fluid retention and controlling problems like ascites in cirrhosis patients makes it critical to recognise high-sodium goods from nutrition labels. People can minimise their salt intake and maintain the health of their liver and overall well-being by making educated selections and comparing the sodium level of each serving to suggested daily limits.

Moreover, reading nutrition labels helps people with cirrhosis determine whether packaged goods contain excessive fats, added sugars, or other potentially harmful ingredients. This well-informed approach to food selection is consistent with the management of cirrhosis, stressing dietary choices that are high in nutrients and favourable to the liver, which help to manage symptoms and improve liver function.

A common misperception about nutrition labels concerns the notion that packaged foods branded as "natural" or "healthy" are automatically in line with the best possible diets. Actually, a thorough examination of the nutrition label is the most effective way to determine the nutritional quality of a food product, as opposed to depending only on marketing claims or the appearance of the packaging to suggest healthfulness. This emphasises how crucial it is to evaluate the veracity of the information included on nutrition labels seriously in order to make educated dietary choices, especially when it comes to controlling cirrhosis and the related nutritional needs.

Ultimately, the capacity to proficiently decipher nutrition labels is a crucial element of successful nutritional management in the setting of cirrhosis. The overall objective of optimising nutrition, controlling symptoms, and promoting liver function can be achieved by people using the information provided on nutrition labels to make health-conscious decisions that are in line with the unique nutritional requirements and limitations associated with cirrhosis.

Lifestyle Modifications

Effective Stress Management

Reducing the detrimental effects of stress on the liver and general health is the aim of appropriate stress management in the setting of cirrhosis. People with cirrhosis can enhance their quality of life and effectively manage their stress by putting into practise tried-and-true methods.

In order to effectively manage stress, people must be open to trying new things, be willing to adapt, and have access to tools like support groups, relaxation techniques, and mental health specialists if necessary.

A multifaceted strategy including lifestyle modifications, relaxation methods, and cognitive-behavioral treatments is necessary for effective stress management. The first step in the process is to comprehend the physiological and psychological consequences that stress has on the body. Next, stress-reduction techniques and habits are put into practise.

1. Understanding Stress and Its Impact on Cirrhosis:

Stress has the potential to worsen cirrhosis symptoms and cause side effects such boosted inflammation, weakened immune system, and liver damage. To properly manage the consequences of stress, one must be aware of its warning signals and how it affects the body.

2. Lifestyle Changes:

- Diet: Stress management requires a healthy, balanced diet. Foods high in nutrients, like fruits, vegetables, whole grains, and lean meats, can improve general health and lessen the negative effects of stress on the body.

- Exercise: Frequent exercise has been demonstrated to lower stress and enhance mental health. For those who have cirrhosis, adding moderate activity to their daily regimen may be helpful.

- Sleep: Getting enough sleep is essential for managing stress. Stress levels can be decreased and sleep quality enhanced by following a regular sleep schedule and soothing nighttime ritual.

3. Relaxation Techniques:

- Deep Breathing: Deep breathing techniques can assist in triggering the relaxation response in the body, which lowers tension and fosters calmness.

- Meditation: It has been demonstrated that practising mindfulness meditation can effectively lower stress and enhance general wellbeing. People can reduce their tension and worry by paying attention to the here and now.

- Progressive Muscle Relaxation: This method encourages both physical and mental relaxation by tensing and then relaxing various bodily muscle groups.

4. Cognitive-Behavioral Strategies:

- Stress Management Training: Acquiring proficient coping mechanisms and problem-solving abilities might enable people to proficiently handle stress and its consequences on their overall welfare.

- Cognitive Restructuring: People can change the way they think and lessen the harmful effects of stress on their mental health by recognising and confronting their negative thought patterns.

It's crucial to speak with a healthcare provider before making any big lifestyle adjustments, particularly when cirrhosis is involved.

- Taking part in stress-relieving hobbies, going out with friends, and spending time in nature can all help manage stress in addition to the other benefits.

- Since alcohol and recreational drugs can worsen the effects of stress on the liver, abstaining from them is imperative.

People can keep an eye on their symptoms, such as better sleep, lower anxiety, and increased general wellbeing, to confirm that stress management is working. Getting input from medical professionals can also validate stress-reduction techniques that work.

When people struggle to put stress management strategies into practise, getting help from mental health specialists, support groups, or internet resources can be a great way to get advice and support.

In summary, a key element in managing cirrhosis is efficient stress management. Through the integration of relaxation techniques, lifestyle modifications, and cognitive-behavioral treatments, people can lessen the detrimental effects of stress on their liver and general health. To ensure that these approaches are successfully implemented, it is crucial to approach stress management as a comprehensive activity, seeking help and direction when needed.

Alcohol and Cirrhosis

Drinking alcohol and being linked to cirrhosis is a serious problem that has to be carefully considered. Alcohol use, especially in excess, has been linked to the onset and advancement of cirrhosis, a chronic liver condition that carries serious health concerns. This chapter will explore the intricate connection between alcohol consumption and cirrhosis. It will also describe the issue, show its effects, present some possible solutions, explain how they would be implemented, and, when appropriate, offer alternatives.

Many cultures have a strong tradition of alcohol usage, which is often included in social events and festive occasions. On the other hand, persistent and heavy alcohol use can harm the liver and cause cirrhosis. Knowing how alcohol affects cirrhosis is important for those who are at risk as well as medical professionals who work with cirrhosis patients.

The main problem is that drinking alcohol is directly linked to the development of cirrhosis. Chronic alcohol misuse can seriously endanger a person's health and well-being by causing liver inflammation, fibrosis, and eventually cirrhosis. It is critical to acknowledge the seriousness of this problem and the possibility that it could harm the liver permanently.

The repercussions of ignoring the issue of excessive alcohol use causing cirrhosis might be severe. Liver failure, portal hypertension, hepatic encephalopathy, and a higher chance of developing liver cancer are all possible outcomes of cirrhosis. It can also have a substantial negative effect on a person's quality of life, resulting in both physical and mental suffering for the afflicted person and their loved ones.

Rehab and alcohol cessation programmes are the most effective ways to treat alcohol-related cirrhosis. These programmes are designed to assist people in cutting back on and eventually quitting alcohol, which can potentially reverse early-stage cirrhosis and stop additional liver damage.

The solution's implementation calls for a multifaceted strategy. It starts with the identification of those who are at risk of developing alcohol-related cirrhosis by means of extensive screening and evaluation. It then involves offering customised interventions, such as behavioural therapy, counselling, and support groups, to help people kick alcohol addiction and make long-lasting lifestyle adjustments.

Comprehensive alcohol cessation programmes, when combined with continued care and monitoring, have the potential to considerably slow the course of cirrhosis and enhance liver function in people with early-stage illness, according to data from prior trials. The expected results indicate that liver fibrosis can regress and the risk of consequences from cirrhosis can be decreased with early management and long-term alcohol abstinence.

Although the main treatment for alcohol-related cirrhosis is quitting alcohol, those who have trouble quitting completely may want to think about harm reduction techniques and medication-assisted therapies. These substitute options must to be thoroughly considered and customised to meet specific requirements, with an emphasis on reducing liver damage and enhancing general health.

In summary, the connection between alcohol use and cirrhosis is a serious problem that calls for an all-encompassing and caring strategy. We may work to lessen the burden of alcohol-related cirrhosis and enhance the lives of those impacted by this complicated disease by understanding the influence of alcohol on liver health, putting effective measures into place, and offering continuing support.

Tobacco and Liver Damage

The use of tobacco and its link to cirrhosis and liver health are important issues that need to be carefully thought out. For ages, people have been consuming tobacco in various ways, and it has been ingrained in many civilizations. However, public health professionals and those at risk of liver disease are very concerned about the effects of smoke on liver health, especially in the context of cirrhosis.

Tobacco usage and liver health are compared in order to shed light on the possible harm that tobacco may do to the liver and to comprehend the complex relationship between tobacco use and the onset and progression of cirrhosis. We hope to clarify the possible dangers and effects of tobacco use on liver health, as well as its implications for those who have cirrhosis, by looking at this comparison.

The physiological effects of tobacco use on the liver, the possible contribution of tobacco use to the onset and progression of cirrhosis, and the distinctions and similarities between alcohol- and tobacco-related liver damage will serve as benchmarks for comparison.

It is clear from comparing alcohol and tobacco usage in terms of liver damage that both can have negative effects on the liver. Tobacco smoke contains a number of harmful substances, including as nicotine and carcinogens, which can cause inflammation and oxidative stress in the liver cells. In a similar vein, long-term alcohol use is linked to liver damage and inflammation, which in turn accelerates the onset of cirrhosis. Their ability to cause liver damage via many methods is what unites them.

Although alcohol and tobacco both have harmful effects on the liver, their mechanisms of action differ greatly from one another. The main distinctions are found in the particular harmful elements of each drug and the ways in which they cause liver damage. For example, the liver's breakdown of alcohol produces harmful byproducts like acetaldehyde that cause direct harm to liver cells, while the components of tobacco, including nitrosamines, can cause DNA damage and encourage mutations in liver cells. Gaining a thorough understanding of these differences is essential to tackling the intricate connection between tobacco use and liver disease.

When comparing the effects of alcohol and tobacco on liver health, using visual aids like charts or diagrams can help the reader better grasp the subtle distinctions between the two substances' effects on the liver and how they may contribute to cirrhosis.

Examining the similarities further highlights the complex relationship between alcohol and tobacco usage and liver impairment. It emphasises the necessity of all-encompassing solutions to address risk factors and the ways in which they affect liver health, especially when cirrhosis is present. Additionally, the analysis clarifies the various mechanisms by which various chemicals might result in liver impairment, highlighting the significance of customised therapies for those afflicted with or at risk for cirrhosis.

By emphasising the continuous public health issues these risk factors represent, tying the comparison of alcohol and tobacco usage to current events might increase relevance. Understanding the unique and overlapping effects of alcohol and tobacco on liver health is crucial in the contemporary context, where the burden of liver disease is still rising, for informing public health policies and individual interventions targeted at reducing the severity and prevalence of cirrhosis.

To sum up, examining the relationship between alcohol and tobacco use and liver damage offers important new perspectives on the complex web of cirrhosis risk factors. By distinguishing the parallels and divergences among these risk variables and their effects on liver function, we can improve our comprehension of the intricate aetiology of cirrhosis and develop efficient management and prophylactic measures.

Weight Management

This chapter's goal is to offer thorough methods for helping people with cirrhosis maintain a healthy weight in order to sustain liver function. The key to controlling cirrhosis and lowering the risk of complications from liver disease is to reach and stay at an ideal body weight.

Seeking advice from a medical expert, such as a liver-health specialist or registered dietician, is crucial prior to starting any weight-management programme. Having access to a range of nutrient-dense foods and being able to exercise are also necessary for putting effective weight management techniques into practise.

For people with cirrhosis, managing their weight is a multifaceted process that includes food adjustments, physical activity, and behavioural changes. The major objective is to get to and stay at a healthy weight that promotes liver function and general wellbeing.

1. It's important to evaluate a person's present weight, body composition, and eating habits before starting any weight-management programme. This could entail taking measurements like the person's waist circumference and body mass index (BMI) in addition to assessing what they typically eat. Knowing current trends is a starting point for creating individualised weight-management plans.

2. People who have cirrhosis frequently have special dietary demands, and depending on the severity of the liver disease and any concomitant issues, different amounts of calories may be needed. A trained dietitian can assist in calculating the right amount of calories consumed and creating a nutritional plan that is balanced and supports liver function in addition to helping with weight management. To achieve critical nutrient requirements, the focus should be on eating nutrient-dense foods such as fruits, vegetables, whole grains, lean meats, and healthy fats.

3. People with cirrhosis benefit from frequent physical activity in terms of managing their weight and general health. An adequate exercise programme should be determined based on the person's medical situation and physical capabilities. This could involve exercises like swimming, walking, or low-impact aerobics that are customised for the person's fitness level and any physical restrictions.

4. Addressing lifestyle variables and behavioural habits that lead to weight fluctuations is a necessary component of sustainable weight management. Techniques including portion control, stress reduction, mindful eating, and creating regular meal schedules can help maintain weight over the long run. Effective weight control also requires addressing any psychological or emotional issues that could affect eating habits.

5. It's critical to regularly check weight, food intake, and physical activity in order to identify progress and make the required modifications to the weight management plan. This could be routine evaluations conducted with a medical expert to determine the efficacy of the tactics used and to make adjustments as necessary to maximise results.

- People with cirrhosis may not benefit from stringent food restrictions or rapid weight loss. Stress the value of making small, lasting changes to help with long-term weight management and reduce the chance of malnutrition.

- Fluid retention is a common symptom of cirrhosis, and abrupt changes in weight may be more indicative of fluid status changes than body fat changes. To properly manage fluid balance, it's critical to keep an eye on fluid intake and collaborate with a healthcare provider.

- Certain drugs that are recommended for the treatment of cirrhosis may have effects on controlling weight. To guarantee comprehensive treatment of the illness, it is crucial to examine any possible interactions or effects on weight with a healthcare professional.

- Because cirrhosis affects the body's ability to absorb nutrients and metabolise them, patients may experience nutritional shortages. Achieving sufficient consumption of vital nutrients, possibly via dietary supplements, might be required to rectify some inadequacies.

Continued assessment of body composition, weight, and pertinent clinical markers can be used to confirm that the weight control plan is being implemented successfully. Furthermore, testing of liver function, energy levels, and general well-being can be used to gauge how well weight management techniques are working.

In the event that people have trouble following the weight-management strategy, it's critical to recognise possible roadblocks and create backup plans. This could entail working through psychological obstacles, getting more help from medical experts, or changing the plan to better suit the requirements and preferences of the individual.

In summary, a customised weight-loss programme is essential for maintaining liver health and improving outcomes for cirrhosis patients. A healthy weight can be attained and maintained by individuals by addressing nutritional, physical, and behavioural aspects that support liver function and general well-being. It's critical to view weight management as a comprehensive undertaking that calls for cooperation with medical specialists and a dedication to long-term, customised plans.

Managing Medications and Toxins

Comprehensive measures to reduce the possibility of worsening liver damage are necessary for the efficient management of cirrhosis. This chapter emphasises the need of abstaining from chemicals that may impair liver function and accelerate the development of cirrhosis, such as medications and toxins. Healthcare practitioners who are involved in the care of persons with cirrhosis must comprehend the effects of different chemicals on liver health. People can improve their general health and proactively support liver function by identifying and reducing potential hazards.

Cirrhosis is an advanced stage of liver disease that is linked to poor liver function and is defined by the increasing scarring of the liver tissue. The liver is especially susceptible to the negative effects of some drugs and pollutants since it is essential to the metabolism of pharmaceuticals and the detoxification of dangerous chemicals. Therefore, in order to protect the health of their livers, people with cirrhosis need to be careful when taking drugs and restrict their exposure to potentially dangerous pollutants.

Because of alterations in drug metabolism and diminished liver function, people with cirrhosis may have problems with their liver's capacity to handle and remove drugs. Some drugs can build up to hazardous amounts in the body, especially those that need hepatic processing, which can have negative side effects and worsen liver damage. Furthermore, exposure to chemicals and pollutants in the environment can put further strain on the liver, which is already impaired, speeding up the advancement of cirrhosis and raising the possibility of consequences.

Take the example of a person who needs pain management due to cirrhosis. Nonsteroidal anti-inflammatory medicines (NSAIDs) like ibuprofen and naproxen can cause gastrointestinal bleeding and damage the liver, especially in people who already have liver disease.

This makes using NSAIDs like these extremely risky. On the other hand, acetaminophen might be a safer option for treating pain in people with cirrhosis if it is used as directed and in moderation.

Moreover, liver function can be severely impacted by exposure to environmental pollutants like alcohol, industrial chemicals, and some herbal medications. Chronic alcohol use, for example, can worsen liver damage and accelerate the development of cirrhosis, which emphasises the need of avoiding alcohol in those with liver disease.

It is critical to understand that the effects of drugs and toxins on liver function might differ depending on the particular cause of the liver disease, the degree of cirrhosis, and the existence of comorbidities in the patient. In addition to taking into account potential interactions and contraindications that may be unique to the patient's medical history and liver function, healthcare professionals must take these factors into account when prescribing medications and counselling patients with cirrhosis on toxin avoidance strategies.

With an estimated incidence of 10–20 percent for hospitalised patients with cirrhosis, the prevalence of adverse medication responses is significantly higher in people with cirrhosis than in the general population. In addition, people with cirrhosis are more vulnerable to drug-induced liver damage, which highlights the importance of careful drug administration and avoidance of toxins in order to protect liver function.

It is crucial to take into account a medicine's hepatic metabolism, potential for drug interactions, and ability to worsen liver injury when assessing possible treatments for people with cirrhosis. Furthermore, being aware of the harmful effects and methods of action of different environmental toxins can enable people to avoid toxins and reduce the chance of further liver damage.

In summary, in order to prevent further liver damage in people with cirrhosis, it is critical to carefully regulate drugs and toxins. Through knowledge of the effects of drugs, poisons, and environmental exposures on liver function, people can protect their liver health in a proactive manner and slow the development of cirrhosis. When it comes to helping patients with cirrhosis make decisions about drug use and toxin avoidance, healthcare providers are essential. This helps patients with cirrhosis receive complete treatment and optimise liver health.

Emotional Well-being and Support

The Psychology of Chronic Illness

Living with cirrhosis involves more than just physical challenges; it also brings with it a host of psychological and emotional challenges that can seriously affect one's overall quality of life. Comprehending these psychological facets is crucial for proficient care of cirrhosis. This chapter delves into the psychology of chronic illness, examining the mental and emotional obstacles that people with cirrhosis may encounter and the methods they employ to manage these complex elements of their health.

Cirrhosis is a chronic illness that can be quite intellectually and emotionally draining to live with. These difficulties must be acknowledged and dealt with since they are critical to a person's general wellbeing. Beyond only the physical symptoms, cirrhosis has a profound psychological impact on all facets of a person's life.

The psychological effects of having cirrhosis are complex. People may feel depressed, anxious, afraid, or that they've lost something because of their health and way of life changing. There might be a heavy psychological cost associated with future uncertainty, possible problems, and the requirement for continuous medical monitoring. The effects of cirrhosis on a person's everyday activities and social relationships may further exacerbate psychological difficulties.

Think about a cirrhosis patient who is constantly anxious about how their illness may worsen and how it will affect their family and work. Their inability to focus and enjoy everyday tasks may be a result of this worry, which may present as a persistent sense of unease. Comprehending these real-world instances aids in appreciating the pragmatic consequences of the psychological obstacles linked to cirrhosis.

It is critical to understand that each person's experience with cirrhosis has a unique psychological impact. When faced with their diagnosis, some people may show extraordinary fortitude and adaptation, while others may find it difficult to handle the emotional and mental toll. Examining these many viewpoints aids in comprehending the complexity of the psychological reactions to long-term disease.

Studies show that those who have cirrhosis have an increased risk of mood disorders such despair and anxiety. Research has indicated that depression symptoms might manifest in as many as 40% of cirrhosis patients, underscoring the substantial psychological impact of the illness. Recognizing the frequency of psychological issues in the management of cirrhosis requires an understanding of these numbers.

It is crucial to define complicated words like psychological resilience, coping strategies, and emotional regulation when talking about the psychology of chronic illness. People can have a better understanding of the psychological processes involved in coping with the difficulties of living with cirrhosis by dissecting these ideas.

Living with cirrhosis presents several psychological difficulties that can seriously lower one's quality of life. It is imperative to acknowledge and tackle these obstacles in order to provide holistic management of cirrhosis. Individuals, caregivers, and medical professionals can create comprehensive plans to assist the psychological health of cirrhosis patients by comprehending the psychological and emotional aspects of the disease.

In conclusion, a crucial component of thorough disease care is understanding the psychology of chronic illness, especially cirrhosis. Through acknowledging and resolving the psychological and emotional obstacles linked to the illness, people might endeavour to improve their general state of health and standard of living. Managing cirrhosis requires a holistic strategy that recognises the complex interactions between mental, emotional, and physical health.

Techniques for Emotional Regulation

This chapter aims to give a thorough overview of emotional regulation approaches that can be applied to manage the psychological effects of cirrhosis and preserve mental equilibrium. Through comprehension and application of these strategies, cirrhosis patients, their family members, and medical professionals can endeavour to improve the mental health and overall standard of living of those impacted by the illness.

The approaches for emotional regulation don't require any special items to be used. However, the effective use of these approaches can be substantially aided by having an open mind, being willing to practise, and having the support of family, friends, and healthcare experts.

A range of behavioural and cognitive techniques are used in emotional regulation to effectively control and cope with emotions. We'll go into great detail on the following strategies: professional counselling, social support, cognitive restructuring, mindfulness and meditation, and relaxation techniques.

1. Being mindful and practising meditation entail paying attention to the here and now while cultivating a non-judgmental awareness of one's thoughts, feelings, and physical sensations. This method helps people to notice their feelings without being sucked into them. Frequent mindfulness and meditation practise has been demonstrated to improve emotional well-being by lowering stress, anxiety, and depressive symptoms.

2. Cognitive restructuring is a treatment approach designed to help patients recognise and confront harmful thought patterns and swap them out for more realistic, balanced ideas. People who have cirrhosis may exhibit cognitive distortions associated with their illness, like overgeneralization or catastrophizing. They can learn to reframe their thoughts and cultivate a more optimistic and adaptable mindset through cognitive restructuring.

3. Various methods of relaxation, such as progressive muscle relaxation, guided visualisation, and deep breathing exercises, can assist people with cirrhosis in stress management and the reduction of emotional excitation. These methods encourage both mental and physical relaxation, which results in a more serene mood and better control over emotions.

4. Using a supportive social network can be very important for managing emotions. Better emotional well-being can be attained by establishing connections with loved ones, friends, support groups, or online communities. These connections can offer a feeling of community, practical guidance, and emotional reassurance.

5. Individuals with cirrhosis can benefit from targeted support for managing the psychological challenges associated with their condition, as well as a safe space to explore their emotions and develop coping mechanisms by seeking professional counselling from psychologists, therapists, or mental health professionals.

It's critical to practise these tactics consistently and to approach them with an open mind. To reap the rewards of emotional management strategies, consistency is essential. Despite their potential for success, these methods cannot replace medical care or expert mental health assistance. People who are in a great deal of mental discomfort ought to get professional assistance.

Research studies and clinical trials have proven the efficacy of these strategies for regulating emotions. The beneficial effects of mindfulness, cognitive restructuring, relaxation methods, social support, and counselling on the emotional well-being of people with chronic illnesses, including cirrhosis, have been shown in several research.

If people have trouble putting these strategies into practise, it could be beneficial to begin with tiny, doable steps and progressively enhance the practise over time. Furthermore, getting advice from medical specialists or mental health specialists can offer individualised support and direction catered to specific need.

To sum up, this chapter's approaches for emotional regulation provide a thorough foundation for managing the psychological effects of cirrhosis and fostering mental equilibrium. People with cirrhosis can improve their general well-being, reduce distress, and develop emotional resilience by adopting these strategies into their daily lives. In order to manage cirrhosis holistically, it is critical to acknowledge the importance of emotional control and to promote its incorporation into all-encompassing care regimens.

Building a Support Network

People with cirrhosis frequently face practical and emotional obstacles as they work through the disease's intricacies, which can have a serious negative influence on their wellbeing. In order to overcome these obstacles, it becomes critical to have a robust support system in place that can provide both practical and emotional help. To promote resilience and improve cirrhosis management, cirrhosis patients, their carers, and medical experts must establish a support system.

For patients and their support networks, cirrhosis can have an unbearable emotional and practical toll. Higher levels of stress, anxiety, and loneliness can result from managing the physical symptoms, treatment plans, and future uncertainty. Without a strong support system, people could find it difficult to adequately manage the complex effects of cirrhosis.

People with cirrhosis may suffer from psychological distress when they don't have a support system, which can worsen their condition and increase their risk of depression, poor treatment compliance, and general health problems. In addition, insufficient assistance might make it difficult to perform everyday responsibilities and medical requirements, exacerbating an already difficult circumstance.

Establishing and utilising a support system provides a proactive way to deal with the psychological and practical difficulties brought on by cirrhosis. People with cirrhosis can become more resilient and better equipped to handle the challenges of their condition by making deep connections and seeking out different kinds of assistance.

Building a support network involves several key steps:

1. People who have cirrhosis should start by determining possible sources of assistance, such as friends, family, support groups, medical experts, and neighbourhood organisations. Identifying the various channels available for seeking assistance is essential to creating a thorough network.

2. It's critical to have effective communication within the support system. Open communication about feelings, worries, and practical needs can help network members become more understanding and empathic. People ought to feel free to express their emotions and ask for help when they need it.

3. It is possible to reduce misunderstandings and encourage positive relationships within the support network by clearly outlining expectations and boundaries. Building a culture of mutual respect and awareness of each person's responsibilities and limitations helps create a peaceful and encouraging atmosphere.

4. Using specialised support services, including social work, counselling, and patient advocacy, can offer assistance that is specifically designed to meet practical and emotional requirements. When it comes to directing people toward pertinent resources and interventions, healthcare professionals are indispensable.

5. People can gain from interacting with online forums, communities, and virtual support groups in the digital age. These networks provide an extra channel for exchanging experiences, getting guidance, and getting emotional support from those going through comparable struggles.

Creating and utilising a support system has been linked to better results for people with cirrhosis and other chronic illnesses. Strong social support has been linked in studies to increased treatment adherence, better coping mechanisms, and psychological well-being. People with cirrhosis can feel empowered and more connected when they actively participate in a support network. This can lead to a more optimistic perspective and an overall higher quality of life.

While creating a support system is a good start, there are other options as well, such as looking into professional care coordination services, participating in peer mentorship programmes, or contacting local groups that support people with chronic illnesses. Cirrhosis management can be optimised by taking into account a diverse approach to support provision and assessing each individual's specific needs.

To sum up, building and utilising a support system is essential to effective cirrhosis management. Through meaningful relationships and collaborative help, people with cirrhosis can overcome their emotional and practical problems and navigate their path with increased resilience and a stronger sense of community. Creating a strong support system is a proactive measure to improve the overall health of individuals with cirrhosis.

Navigating Relationships

Individuals may face difficulties in preserving positive interpersonal relationships while they negotiate the difficulties of managing cirrhosis. Relationships impacted by cirrhosis affect not only the person with the illness but also their friends, family, and caretakers. This case study explores the complexities of relationship management while coping with cirrhosis, highlighting the obstacles, tactics, and results that must be considered.

Following her diagnosis of cirrhosis as a result of nonalcoholic fatty liver disease, 45-year-old Sarah found it difficult to keep the peace in her relationships with others. She had a lot of mental and physical strain from managing her cirrhosis, which made it difficult for her to engage with her spouse, kids, and close friends.

Sarah has always been the pillar of her family—a wonderful wife and mother. David, Sarah's spouse, was encouraging but found it difficult to fully understand the severity of her illness. Jake and Emma, their two teenage children, were struggling with the uncertainties around their mother's diagnosis as well as the changes in their family relationships.

Sarah's main struggle was managing her relationships while dealing with the complex effects of cirrhosis. Her relationships with her family and friends suffered as a result of her physical restrictions, mental anguish, and necessary lifestyle changes. Misunderstandings, poor communication, and unfulfilled expectations added to the difficulties she was facing.

Sarah's healthcare team and she used a multipronged approach to treating her relationship problems, using a range of techniques to build resilience, understanding, and empathy among her support system.

1. Sarah started having frank discussions with her family in which she explained the nature of her illness and how it affected her

day-to-day activities. Within the family, understanding and empathy were based on this open line of communication.

2. In order to deal with the emotional ramifications of her diagnosis, Sarah sought out counselling and psychiatric assistance. She managed the psychological effects of having cirrhosis by learning coping mechanisms under the supervision of a mental health expert, which improved her relationships with her family.

3. Sarah's family members attended informational meetings that her healthcare team and she arranged, giving them thorough details about cirrhosis, its effects, and how they might help her. Giving her family the information they needed to manage Sarah's condition together made them feel more unified and accountable.

4. The family created clear expectations and boundaries for caregiving, emotional support, and practical help through facilitated discussions. This clear definition of duties and responsibilities reduced miscommunication and promoted a positive atmosphere.

The application of these tactics had favourable results in Sarah's connections. Her family's awareness of cirrhosis grew as a result of open conversation and education, which encouraged compassion and support. The dynamic within the family improved as Emma and Jake, Sarah's children, actively participated in her care, and David, her husband, showed increased empathy and support.

The need of proactive communication, knowledge, and psychological support in navigating relationships while controlling cirrhosis is highlighted by this case study. Through addressing the practical and emotional obstacles in her support system, Sarah was able to strengthen her relationships and cultivate resilience, which in turn improved her general well-being.

Visual aids that illustrate the beneficial changes in family dynamics and communication styles when the tactics are put into practise.

Sarah's and her family's experiences highlight the critical role that relationships play in the comprehensive care of cirrhosis. Through fostering compassion, understanding, and support among her network of allies, Sarah not only improved her own wellbeing but also established the groundwork for a strong and resilient family.

What proactive measures can people with cirrhosis do to build resilience and understanding in their relationships with their support systems, which will ultimately help them manage their disease holistically?

In summary, developing strong interpersonal links is crucial for building resilience and maximising well-being as people manage the challenges of cirrhosis. In navigating relationships while managing cirrhosis, this case study highlights the transformational power of proactive communication, education, and psychological support, highlighting their crucial role in the holistic approach to cirrhosis management.

Mindfulness and Meditation

Meditation and mindfulness are becoming more widely acknowledged as effective strategies for enhancing general wellbeing, lowering stress levels, and creating a stronger sense of calm and clarity. When it comes to managing cirrhosis, the application of mindfulness techniques can be a beneficial supplement to therapeutic measures, providing those who have the illness with a comprehensive way to improve their quality of life.

For those with cirrhosis, practising mindfulness and meditation can greatly lower stress, boost emotional health, and improve overall quality of life.

The positive effects of mindfulness and meditation on lowering stress and improving mental health have been shown in several research. Black et al. (2015) observed that individuals with chronic medical problems, such as liver disease, reported feeling less psychologically distressed and having a higher quality of life after using mindfulness-based therapies. Moreover, a meta-analysis conducted by Hilton et al. (2017) demonstrated that mindfulness meditation was useful in lowering anxiety and depressive symptoms across a range of patient demographics, emphasising its possible applicability to people managing long-term medical diseases like cirrhosis.

Numerous processes underlie the beneficial effects of mindfulness and meditation on emotional well-being. Cultivating present-moment awareness, acceptance, and nonjudgmental observation of one's thoughts and emotions are all part of mindfulness practises. People can improve their emotional control and resilience by practising mindfulness meditation, which is especially important when managing a chronic illness like cirrhosis. Studies by Tang et al. (2015) and Hölzel et al. have shown that the practise of mindfulness has been linked to neurobiological changes, including modifications in brain areas involved in emotional processing and control (2011).

In addition, it has been demonstrated that mindfulness training frequently involves the practise of meditation, which triggers physiological relaxation reactions such a drop in blood pressure, heart rate, and cortisol levels, which lessen the physiological effects of stress. Research from Pascoe et al. (2017) and Creswell et al. (2014), which emphasised the benefit of meditation in lowering stress and improving emotional well-being, lends credence to these conclusions.

It's critical to recognise potential obstacles and limitations even in light of the strong evidence for the advantages of mindfulness and meditation. Some opponents contend that individual variations in receptivity and practise adherence may have an impact on the efficacy of mindfulness programmes. To guarantee fair access to and application of these interventions, more research is needed on the accessibility and cultural adaption of mindfulness programmes for a variety of patient populations, including those managing chronic liver illnesses.

Although there may be individual variances in the responsiveness to mindfulness practises, recent studies have highlighted the versatility of mindfulness interventions in a range of contexts and across a variety of populations, including those dealing with long-term health issues. Studies by Lu et al. (2016) and Sauer-Zavala et al. (2016) have demonstrated the potential to engage individuals from a variety of backgrounds using customised mindfulness programmes that take cultural and contextual subtleties into account (2017). These results highlight the potential for mindfulness therapies to promote emotional well-being in a variety of patient populations, including cirrhosis patients, in an inclusive and efficient manner.

Recent research has demonstrated the value of mindfulness and meditation in boosting coping strategies, building resilience, and encouraging self-care among people with chronic health issues, which adds to the body of data demonstrating these practises' positive effects. A study conducted in 2010 by Matousek et al. showed that mindfulness-based stress reduction improves coping mechanisms and lowers psychological distress in patients with chronic illnesses, indicating that it may be useful in the treatment of cirrhosis.

In summary, the integration of mindfulness and meditation techniques exhibits significant potential for mitigating stress, improving psychological health, and elevating the general standard of living for cirrhosis patients. The growing body of research demonstrating the positive effects of mindfulness therapies and the increasing flexibility of these techniques in a variety of patient populations highlights their potential as useful supplements to all-encompassing cirrhosis management approaches. Healthcare professionals and patients with cirrhosis can develop a comprehensive strategy for fostering resilience and well-being in the face of chronic illness by including mindfulness and meditation into the treatment continuum.

Counseling and Therapy

In order to provide people with the full care they need to navigate the many obstacles that come with having cirrhosis, counselling and therapy are essential. Healthcare professionals, patients, and their families must comprehend the key words involved in counselling and therapy in order to interact with the material and appreciate the importance of these interventions in the treatment of cirrhosis.

The following terminology will be defined and discussed in order to help promote a structured and clear understanding of counselling and therapy in the context of managing cirrhosis:

1. Counseling
2. Therapy
3. Psychotherapy
4. Behavioral Therapy
5. Support Groups
6. Cognitive-Behavioral Therapy (CBT)
7. Family Therapy
8. Coping Strategies
9. Emotional Regulation
10. Resilience

1. A qualified counsellor or therapist works in tandem with a person who has cirrhosis to provide counselling in the context of managing the disease. It includes a variety of supportive interventions designed to address social, psychological, and emotional issues. It offers a secure environment in which patients can discuss their experiences, feelings, and ideas regarding their disease. The goals of counselling are to improve coping mechanisms, support mental health, and enable well-informed choices about the management of cirrhosis.

2. The term "therapy" refers to a wider range of interventions intended to address the psychological and emotional difficulties that people with cirrhosis face. The strategy comprises many evidence-based

methods customised to meet the specific requirements of each person, with the ultimate objective of fostering mental well-being, adaptability, and resilience. Individual, group, and family therapy are all possible, and certified mental health professionals—such as psychologists, social workers, and counselors—are frequently the ones who provide it.

3. Psychotherapy is the application of psychological concepts and techniques to assist patients in navigating relationships with others, managing emotional discomfort, and creating coping mechanisms for the effects of cirrhosis on their lives. It includes a broad spectrum of therapeutic methods, each specifically designed to address different facets of an individual's emotional and psychological well-being, such as cognitive-behavioral therapy, psychodynamic therapy, and humanistic approaches.

4. The goal of behavioural therapy is to recognise and alter maladaptive habits of behaviour and thinking that could exacerbate discomfort or make it more difficult to effectively manage cirrhosis. It is based on learning theory concepts and seeks to improve self-regulation, encourage positive behavioural change, and lessen the negative effects of psychological factors on an individual's general well-being.

5. Support groups offer a vital forum for people with cirrhosis to interact with others going through comparable struggles, exchange stories, and get educational and emotional support. These support groups, which can be led by peer leaders or medical experts, provide a feeling of belonging, validation, and encouragement. They also provide a network of people who can help each other deal with the emotional and social challenges of having cirrhosis.

6. Cognitive Behavioral Therapy (CBT) is a goal-oriented, structured type of psychotherapy that aims to promote adaptive coping and emotional regulation by recognising and changing harmful thought patterns and actions. It highlights the relationship between ideas, feelings, and actions and gives people useful tools to handle the stress, worry, and despair that are frequently brought on by cirrhosis.

7. Family therapy acknowledges how cirrhosis affects the entire family and how familial relationships are intertwined. It seeks to address family communication styles, interpersonal issues, and coping mechanisms in order to create a nurturing atmosphere that enhances the wellbeing of the cirrhosis patient and their loved ones.

8. Coping strategies include the adaptive mechanisms and methods people use to deal with the practical and emotional difficulties brought on by cirrhosis. To boost psychological health and resilience, these tactics could involve seeking out social support, practising emotion management, problem-solving approaches, and participating in worthwhile activities.

9. The capacity to control and adjust one's emotional reactions to stressors, difficulties, and life events is known as emotional regulation. For people with cirrhosis, emotional regulation is essential because it can reduce the severity of emotional distress, improve decision-making, and encourage flexible coping mechanisms in the face of the condition's complications.

10. The ability to adjust and prosper in the midst of hardship is referred to as resilience. It is the culmination of both internal and external resources that help people overcome the obstacles that come with having cirrhosis. Resilience is the capacity to recover from setbacks, hold onto a sense of meaning and optimism, and develop flexible coping mechanisms that promote psychological health.

Making connections between these concepts and actual events helps clarify their meaning and encourage in-depth contemplation. Think about the feelings of a person with cirrhosis who is more anxious and worried about their health in the future. Through counselling, this person can talk openly about their anxieties, feel supported and validated, and regain control over their emotional health. During treatment, patients might acquire cognitive-behavioral methods to confront destructive thought patterns, fostering emotional control and resilience similar to creating a mental "toolbox" for dealing with the difficulties brought on by cirrhosis.

Family therapy recognises the interdependence of familial support and the necessity for a strong foundation to withstand the storms of cirrhosis, much like tending to a tree's roots. Support groups can be likened to a communal garden, where people come together to share their experiences, offer support in the form of empathy and understanding, and work together to build hope and resilience in the face of hardship.

These real-world examples highlight the potential of counselling and therapy to support emotional well-being, adaptive coping, and resilience in the lives of those living with cirrhosis, and they also serve to highlight the practical implications of these interventions in the context of managing the chronic illness.

This material offers a thorough grasp of the critical role that therapy and counselling play in managing cirrhosis, giving patients, caregivers, and healthcare professionals the information and understanding they need to interact with these crucial interventions in an efficient manner.

Coping With Grief and Loss

Because cirrhosis has such a profound effect on people's life, dealing with grief and loss is a crucial part of treating the disease for both the affected person and their loved ones. The psychological effects of cirrhosis can include anxiety about the future, changes in lifestyle, and bereavement over health loss. This can lead to a complicated emotional landscape that requires specialised care and management. For the purpose of successfully navigating and addressing the emotional aspects of this chronic condition, healthcare professionals, patients, and their families must comprehend the complex nature of grieving and its implications in the context of cirrhosis.

The main problem here is that cirrhosis has a tremendous emotional impact, especially when it comes to loss and mourning. People who have cirrhosis frequently experience the loss of their prior level of freedom, health, and way of life, which can cause severe bereavement. Additionally, as they face the difficulties of helping their loved ones navigate the complexity of cirrhosis, family members and caregivers may suffer from anticipatory grieving. If left untreated, grief and loss can seriously worsen emotional discomfort, jeopardise mental health, and make it more difficult for patients and their support systems to effectively manage cirrhosis.

There are numerous negative effects that might arise if the emotional impact of cirrhosis—specifically, loss and grief—is not recognised and addressed. People may endure protracted emotional anguish, elevated anxiety, sadness, and a feeling of loneliness, all of which can have a negative effect on their general quality of life. Unresolved loss and grief can also make it more difficult to develop healthy coping mechanisms, intensify interpersonal disputes, and create the supportive networks that are essential for managing cirrhosis. Moreover, the cumulative effects of untreated emotional distress can worsen medical symptoms, impair treatment compliance, and jeopardise the general wellbeing of people living with cirrhosis.

A comprehensive strategy for managing loss and sorrow in the setting of cirrhosis entails putting into practise focused interventions intended to enhance resilience, encourage adaptive coping, and support emotional well-being. This can include a multifaceted approach that combines psychoeducation, individual and group therapy techniques, and the development of a framework for a supportive community. Through the recognition and management of bereavement and loss, patients and the people who support them can build the emotional fortitude required to effectively and psychologically manage the intricacies of cirrhosis.

A comprehensive strategy that includes individual counselling, group therapy, and psychoeducational programmes catered to the specific requirements of people and their families is required for the implementation of a grieving and loss intervention framework. In order to address sorrow and loss in the context of cirrhosis, mental health professionals—such as licenced counsellors, psychologists, and social workers—can play a critical role in offering focused support, psychoeducation, and evidence-based therapy therapies. Furthermore, combining peer support groups with community-based services can give people a forum to interact, exchange stories, and get encouragement and validation—all of which can promote a feeling of resilience and support among the group as a whole.

Targeted grieving and loss therapies are effective in fostering emotional well-being and adaptive coping mechanisms in people with cirrhosis, according to empirical data and clinical insights. Studies have indicated that comprehensive bereavement and loss therapies can decrease feelings of anxiety, despair, and emotional distress while also improving people's resilience, sense of community, and general quality of life. Through proactive grieving and loss management, patients and their support systems can develop the emotional fortitude required to effectively and psychologically manage the complications of cirrhosis.

When examining other options, it's critical to acknowledge the benefits of complementary strategies like expressive therapy, mindfulness-based interventions, and cognitive-behavioral methods designed to deal with loss and grieving in the context of cirrhosis. These methods can provide people with extra resources to help them manage their emotional suffering, develop self-awareness, and create flexible coping mechanisms. Furthermore, the inclusion of family therapy can offer a complete approach to supporting cirrhosis patients and their loved ones through the complex stages of grieving and loss. Family therapy focuses on addressing the impact of cirrhosis on the entire family unit.

In summary, the psychological effects of cirrhosis, especially when it comes to loss and grieving, provide a serious obstacle that calls for specialised care and assistance. Through the recognition and management of the intricacies associated with bereavement and loss, people and the others who support them can develop the emotional fortitude required to effectively and psychologically manage the complicated obstacles associated with cirrhosis. In the face of this chronic condition, people with cirrhosis and their loved ones can promote adaptive coping techniques, emotional well-being, and collective resilience by putting into practise evidence-based grief and loss interventions and incorporating supportive community frameworks.

Planning for the Future

Understanding Prognosis

A chronic, progressive liver condition called cirrhosis causes scar tissue to gradually replace healthy liver tissue until liver failure occurs. Patients with cirrhosis and those who care for them must be aware of the prognosis in order to make decisions about therapy and way of life. This chapter will examine the intricacies surrounding the prognosis of cirrhosis, including the different elements that impact long-term results and successful management techniques.

Based on the unique circumstances of each patient and the state of medical knowledge at the time of diagnosis, prognosis describes the expected trajectory and result of a disease, in this case cirrhosis. It entails determining the extent of the liver damage, whether complications are present, and how well the treatment is working. Individual differences in the degree of liver damage, the underlying aetiology of the disease, and the existence of comorbidities can all have a significant impact on the prognosis of cirrhosis.

In order to clarify the meaning of prognosis in cirrhosis, let's look at a fictitious case study. A 55-year-old male patient named Patient A has severe cirrhosis and a history of alcohol misuse. Patient A has growing liver dysfunction and develops problems such ascites and hepatic encephalopathy even after undergoing treatment and following lifestyle changes, including quitting alcohol. Patient B, a 45-year-old woman with non-alcoholic fatty liver disease, on the other hand, makes lifestyle adjustments and is routinely monitored, which leads to the stabilisation of her liver function and the avoidance of problems. These opposing situations demonstrate how different factors can have an impact on cirrhosis prognosis.

When assessing the prognosis of cirrhosis, it is imperative to take into account multiple viewpoints. Medical experts use clinical signs like the Child-Pugh score and the Model for End-Stage Liver Disease (MELD) score to determine the severity of liver disease. These instruments aid in prognosis-based patient stratification and direct therapeutic choices. In addition, patients' and their families' opinions on the course of the disease and its effects on their lives may be distinct according to their own experiences, convictions, and expectations.

A thorough grasp of the prognosis for cirrhosis necessitates the inclusion of pertinent facts and statistics. The American Liver Foundation estimates that within ten years, thirty percent of patients with compensated cirrhosis will develop decompensated cirrhosis, while fifty percent of patients with decompensated cirrhosis survive for ten years. These figures highlight how cirrhosis progresses and how it has a major influence on long-term results.

Many technical words and medical jargon may come up when discussing the prognosis of cirrhosis, which could be confusing to patients and their families. For example, phrases like "variceal haemorrhage," "portal hypertension," and "hepatocellular carcinoma" are frequently linked to issues related to cirrhosis. People can better understand the effects of these medical problems on their prognosis and overall management if these terms are clarified and simplified.

In summary, there are several facets to comprehending the prognosis of cirrhosis, including practical, psychological, and medical aspects. With a thorough evaluation of the severity of liver disease, customised case management, and integration of supportive care, patients and healthcare providers can work together to effectively manage the difficulties related to the prognosis of cirrhosis. In the end, cirrhosis patients' quality of life and long-term results can be improved by arming people with information and proactive management techniques.

We will go into more detail about many facets of managing cirrhosis in the upcoming chapters, such as lifestyle changes, therapeutic options, and the all-encompassing strategy for improving the quality of life for cirrhosis patients.

Advanced Directives and Planning

The significance of advanced directives and planning in the treatment of cirrhosis cannot be emphasised. People may have to make difficult medical decisions and think about end-of-life care as the illness worsens. Advanced directives provide patients the ability to specify their choices for medical interventions and choose a reliable person to make healthcare decisions on their behalf in the event of an incapacitating illness. These documents include living wills and healthcare proxies. In addition to medical emergencies, planning for cirrhosis involves making mental and practical arrangements to enhance the lives of patients and their families.

Informed decisions and moral conundrums in healthcare decision-making can result from the absence of detailed planning and prior directives in the management of cirrhosis. Medical professionals may encounter difficulties matching treatments to a patient's values and objectives if they do not receive clear direction from patients regarding their preferences for their course of care. Proactive planning can also help reduce stress and emotional strain for caregivers and family members, who may find it difficult to make tough decisions without the patient's input.

If people with cirrhosis fail to participate in advanced directives and planning, there could be serious repercussions. Lack of specific directions may cause lengthy decision-making procedures in the event of a medical emergency, such as acute decompensation or the necessity for liver transplantation, which would increase the patient's and their family's stress and anxiety. Furthermore, in the absence of a named healthcare proxy, the burden of making important medical decisions could fall on those who are not entirely cognizant of the patient's desires, which could result in a discrepancy between the treatment received and the patient's requests.

The proactive management of the complications associated with cirrhosis can be achieved by the combination of advanced directives and extensive planning. People can express their beliefs, treatment choices, and end-of-life care concerns by having meaningful conversations with loved ones and healthcare professionals. Patients can choose a reliable advocate to make sure their healthcare choices follow their wishes even if they are unable to express them directly by setting up a healthcare proxy.

There are numerous critical steps in the application of advanced directives and planning for the management of cirrhosis. First and foremost, patients should have candid discussions about their goals of care, including their preferences for palliative care, end-of-life interventions, and life-sustaining therapies, with their healthcare team. Afterwards, people can put their decisions into legal form by drafting enforceable agreements that specify their healthcare preferences and name a proxy for them, such as living wills and durable powers of attorney for healthcare. It is essential that these directives be reviewed and updated on a frequent basis to account for any modifications to the patient's personal beliefs or medical status.

Research indicates that the application of advanced directives and extensive planning in the management of cirrhosis results in increased patient satisfaction, less healthcare expenses, and better match between patient wishes and medical interventions. Knowing that their healthcare decisions are recorded and upheld gives people who participate in advance care planning a sense of empowerment and peace of mind. In addition, the presence of a designated healthcare proxy ensures that the patient's wishes are honoured across the care continuum by facilitating more effective communication between healthcare practitioners and the patient's support system.

While planning and advanced directives are essential to the management of cirrhosis, in some cases, other options can also be worth taking into account. Advanced directives can be augmented by the inclusion of interdisciplinary care teams and supportive services, such as social workers and palliative care specialists, for individuals who struggle with decision-making because of cognitive impairment or lack of social support. Furthermore, patient and family decision-making can be encouraged to be proactive and well-informed through training programmes designed to increase knowledge of advance care planning in the cirrhosis community.

In summary, the incorporation of comprehensive planning and advanced directives into the management of cirrhosis forms the basis of patient-centered care, fostering dignity, autonomy, and well-informed decision-making. People with cirrhosis and their families can manage the intricacies of the disease with clarity and confidence by proactively addressing end-of-life care considerations and communicating treatment preferences. This helps to promote a compassionate and controllable healthcare journey. We will explore useful approaches to starting conversations about advance care planning and negotiating the moral issues surrounding the treatment of cirrhosis in the upcoming chapters.

Insurance and Financial Planning

This chapter aims to give readers a thorough understanding of insurance and financial planning as crucial elements of managing cirrhosis. Through the clear explanation of the required actions and factors, readers will be able to handle the intricacies of insurance plans and budgetary planning, guaranteeing the best possible access to medical care and reducing the financial strain related to cirrhosis treatment.

Prior to discussing insurance and budgeting for the management of cirrhosis, people should make sure they have all the relevant data they need, such as financial accounts, medical expense records, and current insurance plans. It will also be easier to grasp the ideas covered in this chapter if you have a basic awareness of financial concepts and insurance terminology.

Insurance and budgeting for the treatment of cirrhosis involve a complex strategy to protect patients from the financial consequences of the illness. This include assessing current insurance coverage, looking into opportunities for supplemental insurance, and putting sensible financial plans in place to deal with any prospective costs related to cirrhosis therapy. People can maximise their access to necessary healthcare services and financial readiness by methodically navigating this process.

1. - Examine existing health insurance plans to find out what services, such as hospital stays, prescription drugs, diagnostic testing, and specialist consultations, are covered for cirrhosis.

- Examine the insurance policies' exclusions and restrictions to find any possible coverage gaps that would need for more insurance or other forms of alternative funding.

2. - To enhance the coverage offered by current health insurance policies, look into the availability of additional insurance plans, such as long-term care insurance or critical illness insurance.

- To choose the best coverage for cirrhosis-related needs, weigh the advantages, restrictions, and financial costs of several supplemental insurance choices.

3. - Create a detailed budget that accounts for all expected costs associated with cirrhosis, such as prescription drugs, hospital stays, medical consultations, and diagnostic tests.

- Use budgeting techniques to set aside money for medical expenses, making sure that the most important medical services are covered first in the overall financial plan.

4. - Examine the use of HSAs and FSAs to reserve pre-tax money for eligible medical costs; this offers a tax-favored way to pay for cirrhosis-related medical costs.

5. - Seek advice from insurance and financial consultants who specialise in healthcare planning to learn about customised insurance plans and financial strategies that are appropriate for managing cirrhosis.

- Tip 1: Examine insurance plans proactively once a year to make sure that the coverage complies with changing medical requirements and any adjustments to the treatment of cirrhosis.

- Tip 2: Examine the potential for government- or employer-sponsored group insurance plans or healthcare initiatives to augment private insurance coverage for cirrhosis-related services.

- Warning: Insufficient insurance coverage and inadequate financial preparation might result in significant out-of-pocket costs and obstacles to receiving necessary cirrhosis therapies, which could jeopardise the disease's overall management.

The effectiveness of insurance and financial planning techniques can be verified by conducting a thorough evaluation of insurance coverage, creating a well-organized budget for cirrhosis-related costs, and consulting a specialist to maximise insurance and financial arrangements.

If people have trouble understanding insurance coverage or coming up with appropriate financial plans, patient advocacy groups, financial counsellors, and medical professionals can help people work through complicated insurance and financial planning problems.

A comprehensive approach to managing cirrhosis with financial stability and resilience can be fostered by individuals who proactively mitigate the disease's economic impact and maximise their access to necessary healthcare services by attending to insurance and financial planning in the context of cirrhosis management. We will cover other aspects of managing cirrhosis in the upcoming chapters, including lifestyle changes, medical interventions, and psychosocial support to help people on their path to overall well-being while living with cirrhosis.

Employment and Cirrhosis

As we go deeper into the intricate world of managing cirrhosis, it becomes critical to discuss the important connection between the consequences of this chronic illness and work. Employment and cirrhosis have a complex link that extends beyond the mental and physical difficulties that people with the disease experience to include the ethical and legal issues that support their rights and obligations at work. We will take a thorough look at the dynamics at work in this chapter, explaining the difficulties, approaches, and results of managing work life while sick. By doing this, we hope to equip people with the information and resources they need to successfully negotiate this complex landscape and promote a comprehensive strategy for managing cirrhosis that takes into account their health, work, and overall well-being.

First, let's set the scene for our case study. Examine the case of Mr. James, a 45-year-old man whose persistent hepatitis C infection resulted in cirrhosis diagnosis. For more than ten years, Mr. James has been a devoted worker at a respectable financial company. He currently has a managerial role that entails active participation in high-pressure decision-making and leadership duties. His physical endurance has been greatly affected by his cirrhosis diagnosis, which has led to weariness, sporadic nausea, and a decreased capacity for sustained periods of concentrated concentration and cognitive sharpness.

The main character of this case study, Mr. James, stands in for the broad group of people who must strike a delicate balance between their obligations to their jobs and the difficulties brought on by cirrhosis. Furthermore, his company, the HR division, and his coworkers are important characters in the storey, each offering unique viewpoints and consequences to the dynamics of work in the context of cirrhosis.

The main difficulty is balancing the physical constraints of cirrhosis with the demands of the workplace. Mr. James faces the difficult challenge of managing the symptoms and limitations of his illness while retaining his professional effectiveness. In addition, he must confront the difficult task of telling his boss and coworkers about his cirrhosis diagnosis. He worries about the possible fallout from stigma or false beliefs about chronic illnesses in the workplace.

In order to tackle these issues, Mr. James starts a multifaceted, all-encompassing strategy. In order to discuss the Americans with Impairments Act (ADA) and its rules about reasonable accommodations for those with disabilities, including those who have chronic diseases like cirrhosis, he first sets up a private meeting with the human resources department. Then, he works with his medical social worker and hepatologist to create a customised plan that incorporates energy-saving techniques, lifestyle changes, and flexible work schedules to maximise his productivity at work while addressing the constraints presented by cirrhosis.

Mr. James's proactive approach has produced a variety of results. He successfully negotiates a modified work schedule that provides flexible hours and the ability to work from home when needed by being transparent and cooperative with his employer. Furthermore, his firm offers ergonomic accommodations to lessen the physical strain that comes with extended desk-based employment, such as an adjustable workstation and supportive seats. Despite the difficulties created by cirrhosis, Mr. James's work productivity and job satisfaction significantly improve as a result, creating an environment that is favourable for professional progress and fulfilment.

The present case study provides significant insights into the critical functions of anticipatory communication, legal acumen, and cooperative problem-solving techniques in effectively managing the intricate interplay between employment and cirrhosis. It emphasises how important it is for people who have cirrhosis to speak up for themselves and have honest conversations with their employers in order to create a welcoming and inclusive workplace. It also emphasises the possible benefits of flexible work schedules and acceptable adjustments for improving the stability and well-being of professionals who are managing cirrhosis at work.

Given this, a chart outlining the range of ADA-required reasonable accommodations for people with cirrhosis could be a useful visual assistance in explaining the many approaches that can be taken to maximise workplace accessibility and functionality for people with chronic diseases.

Mr. James's experiences are a microcosm of the larger storey about the inclusion of people with long-term illnesses in the labour. Employers may capitalise on the tremendous potential of people living with cirrhosis by creating a culture of awareness, empathy, and proactive support. This will help to create a more diverse and equitable workplace.

As we come to the end of this case study, it makes us think about how organisational rules and legal frameworks affect how people with chronic illnesses interact at work. How can legislators and businesses work together to improve the support networks and accessibility that people with cirrhosis and other chronic illnesses have in the workplace?

We will explore further aspects of managing cirrhosis in the upcoming chapters, including psychological fortitude, social networks, and lifestyle adjustments to provide people with comprehensive tools for coping with the challenges of living with cirrhosis.

Home and Health Adaptations

As we traverse the complex terrain of managing cirrhosis, it is critical to acknowledge the significant influence that health and home modifications can have on the health and well-being of those living with this long-term illness. Living space and routine adjustments are an important part of cirrhosis management; they provide a multimodal way to lessen the logistical, emotional, and physical difficulties associated with the disease. This chapter will include a thorough examination of the adaptive methods that can be used to optimise daily routines and the home environment, creating a setting that supports the comfort, safety, and functional independence of people with cirrhosis.

a. The cornerstone of managing cirrhosis in the home is the use of ergonomic adjustments that address the particular physical requirements and constraints imposed by this illness. This includes placing appliances and furniture in a way that reduces physical strain, installing grab bars and handrails to help with mobility and stability, and optimising lighting to lessen the effects of visual disturbances that may come with cirrhosis-related complications like hepatic encephalopathy.

b. The relationship between nutrition and the management of cirrhosis highlights how important dietary changes are for maintaining liver function and reducing cirrhosis symptoms. People who have cirrhosis are frequently recommended to follow a low-sodium diet in order to reduce fluid retention. It is also important to make sure that they get enough protein in order to prevent malnourishment and muscular atrophy. In addition, incorporating nutrient-dense foods—like fruits, vegetables, and whole grains—is essential to nutritional optimization because it promotes a well-rounded, nourishing diet that benefits liver function and general wellbeing.

c. One important aspect of managing cirrhosis is incorporating customised physical activity regimens, which have positive effects on the functional, psychological, and physiological domains. Low-impact workouts, such swimming, walking, or stationary cycling, are recommended for people with cirrhosis in order to preserve muscle mass, improve cardiovascular fitness, and lessen the physical deconditioning that can result from fatigue and inactivity related to the disease. Furthermore, exercise is a powerful means of enhancing mental health by creating a feeling of confidence and success despite the difficulties associated with cirrhosis.

d. Attention, memory, and executive function deficiencies are among the cognitive symptoms of cirrhosis that highlight the need for focused therapies to improve cognitive function at home. Puzzles, word games, and memory drills are examples of cognitive exercises that are useful for maintaining cognitive function and promoting brain plasticity. This helps to lessen the negative effects of hepatic encephalopathy and cognitive impairment on day-to-day functioning and quality of life.

e. The emotional aspects of managing cirrhosis require an all-encompassing strategy that includes developing emotional resilience, reducing stress and anxiety, and managing emotional instability that may arise from difficulties associated to the disease. Relaxation methods, cognitive-behavioral approaches, and mindfulness-based practises are effective ways to promote emotional well-being in the home, enabling people with cirrhosis to deal with the emotional upheaval that comes with their chronic illness with strength and grace.

f. Establishing strong social support networks in the home is a vital component of the all-encompassing care of cirrhosis patients. It provides opportunities for social interaction, practical help, and emotional support that can significantly improve the quality of life for those living with this illness. The cornerstones of social support are family, friends, and support groups. They offer channels for compassion, understanding, and companionship that can lessen feelings of loneliness and isolation that may arise from managing cirrhosis.

g. To maximise therapeutic outcomes and prevent potential consequences, the complexities of hydration and drug management in the home setting require a careful strategy that include compliance, attentiveness, and education. A proactive and empowered approach to fluid and medication management in the home environment is fostered by the advice given to people with cirrhosis to monitor their fluid intake, follow prescribed medication regimens, and promptly report any signs of medication-related adverse effects or disease progression to their healthcare providers.

The incorporation of these adaptive measures into the home setting constitutes a comprehensive strategy for managing cirrhosis that balances the domains of physical, psychological, and practical well-being. Through the cultivation of a home environment that is sensitive to the distinct requirements and obstacles presented by cirrhosis, individuals can enhance their resilience and strengthen their ability to manage the intricacies of living with the disease. As we explore the real-world uses of these adaptable tactics, we will highlight the significant influence they can have on improving the standard of living and overall health for those navigating the challenging terrain of managing cirrhosis.

Community and Government Resources

Navigating the complex support and resource environment in the field of cirrhosis management is essential to developing a holistic approach that takes into account the logistical, psychological, and physical aspects of this chronic illness. Resources from the community and the government are priceless tools that may help people living with cirrhosis and those who care for them feel resilient, empowered, and holistically well. This chapter begins with a critical examination of the wide range of community and governmental services that are accessible to people who have cirrhosis, explaining their functions and outlining their significant consequences for the best possible management of the disease.

Community resources comprise an array of regional programmes, associations, and assistance systems specifically designed to cater to the particular requirements of cirrhosis patients. These resources can include advocacy groups, counselling services, educational courses, and support groups. Their goal is to give cirrhosis patients and their families a caring and compassionate environment. Government resources, on the other hand, comprise the range of public assistance programmes, healthcare services, and legislative provisions that are intended to provide real support and advocacy for people who have cirrhosis. These programmes address the medical, financial, and social needs of these individuals within the framework of larger public welfare initiatives.

The variety of community resources is what makes them so unique; they include a wide range of programmes and services that address the complex requirements of people living with cirrhosis. Through platforms for practical advice, emotional support, and companionship, support groups and counselling programmes give people with cirrhosis and those who care for them a sense of community, empathy, and understanding amongst the difficulties this chronic condition presents. In order to promote knowledge, understanding, and social change, advocacy groups and educational seminars act as channels for information dissemination, empowering, and amplifying the voices of people living with cirrhosis in the larger public conversation.

Conversely, government resources have a unique effect because of their institutional foundation and legal requirements. For people with cirrhosis, public support programs—disability benefits, healthcare subsidies, housing aid—act as lifelines by reducing financial pressures and guaranteeing access to necessary medical care and housing. In addition, legislation and regulations pertaining to disability rights, anti-discrimination, and healthcare reforms act as strongholds for advocacy and protection, preserving the rights, dignity, and general welfare of people with cirrhosis within the framework of public welfare and societal governance.

The way that government and community resources have changed in the context of managing cirrhosis is indicative of a paradigm shift in how chronic illness and disability are perceived and treated. In the past, people who had cirrhosis faced significant obstacles when trying to obtain all the resources and assistance they needed. They also had to deal with stigma, social exclusion, and institutionalised neglect, which made their disease even more difficult to manage. But a transformative renaissance in the availability of resources and support for people with cirrhosis has been sparked by the growth of patient advocacy movements, the emergence of community-based initiatives, and the passing of disability rights legislation. This has ushered in a new era of societal recognition, empowerment, and inclusion for this population.

Resources provided by the community and the government are important not just for the individual but also for the welfare, advocacy, and public health of society as a whole. These resources create a societal ethos of empathy, inclusion, and equity by supporting a supportive ecosystem that enhances the resilience and well-being of people with cirrhosis. This lays the foundation for a more understanding and compassionate society that upholds the rights and dignity of people with chronic conditions. Additionally, government and community resources act as catalysts for systemic change by elevating the voices and experiences of people living with cirrhosis and supporting legislative changes, advancements in healthcare, and social programmes that support the values of justice, accessibility, and dignity for all citizens.

The concrete influence of governmental and community resources is evident in the lives of people living with cirrhosis, significantly influencing their experiences, adaptability, and general well-being. Support organisations, such the "Cirrhosis Care Coalition" and the "Liver Health Alliance," give people with cirrhosis a forum to talk about their experiences, learn from peers, and get emotional support and advice from those who have faced comparable obstacles. In addition, these organisations provide social gatherings, caregiver workshops, and educational seminars to promote understanding and solidarity among people with cirrhosis.

Government programmes like the Medicaid waiver for home and community-based services and the Supplemental Security Income (SSI) programme provide individuals with cirrhosis with critical financial assistance and healthcare coverage. These resources guarantee that these individuals have access to critical medical care, medications, and supportive services that are critical to their well-being and ability to function independently. Furthermore, legal provisions like the Patient Protection and Affordable Care Act (ACA) and the Americans with Disabilities Act (ADA) have sparked enormous progress in defending the rights, accessibility, and dignity of people with cirrhosis, promoting a climate of social inclusion, equity, and empowerment.

The profound relevance of community and government resources in the context of cirrhosis management may be obscured by widespread misconceptions and misinterpretations, despite the resources' transforming impact. A common misperception is that people living with cirrhosis should only depend on medical treatments and family support. This ignores the vital role that government and community resources play in promoting advocacy, empowerment, and social inclusion for people with this condition. Furthermore, people with cirrhosis may be discouraged from pursuing necessary public assistance programmes and services due to the false belief that accessing government resources is difficult and time-consuming. This could result in continued financial hardships and healthcare disparities that could be avoided by making proactive use of these resources.

In summary, government and community resources are the cornerstones of social advocacy, empowerment, and support for people with cirrhosis, enhancing their journeys with dignity, resiliency, and understanding. People with cirrhosis and those who care for them can create a path of empowerment, inclusion, and overall well-being by utilising the diverse range of community and government resources that are available. This allows them to overcome the obstacles that this chronic illness presents and create lives that are full of hope, support, and social recognition.

Creating a Legacy

With the gentle afternoon light streaming through the transparent curtains, I sat in my office and thought about all the inspiring tales of hope and resiliency that had passed through this room over the years. I was particularly struck by a storey that captured the spirit of the cirrhosis journey, which is one that is full of obstacles but is also characterised by the resolute determination of people who must traverse its treacherous path.

When I first met Mr. and Mrs. Patel, a couple whose life had been drastically changed by the diagnosis of cirrhosis, it was a cool autumn morning. The smell of earthy fallen leaves filled the air, as a little breeze rustled the tree branches outside my window, reflecting the room's shifting emotional tides.

Mr. Patel was a retired teacher with a soft spoken, placid strength that belied the conflict inside. He loved to tell stories. The artist Mrs. Patel exuded a lively personality that was evident in her works, and her graceful demeanour concealed the uncertainty that loomed large in their life.

Every piece of their storey came to life like a tapestry of feelings and encounters, creating a striking picture of resiliency and willpower in the face of difficulty. Their tale skillfully woven a tapestry of human strength and fragility, from the initial shock of the diagnosis to the maze-like complexity of therapy and care.

Their eyes revealed the hidden anxieties that were there, and their voices trembled with a strong mixture of hope and terror. The real scope of their battle emerged during those exposed times of vulnerability, going beyond the clinical confines of their illness to include the deep emotional and psychological aspects of their journey.

But in the middle of their story's turmoil, something unexpected happened—a turn that would completely change the way they saw life, meaning, and legacy. They found an unwavering tenacity, a creative wellspring, and a profound sense of interconnectedness with the world around them in the furnace of their battle.

Despite being extremely personal, their narrative struck a chord with universal truths that go beyond the boundaries of disease and misfortune. It discussed the resiliency of people, the transformational potential of art, and the enduring legacy of love and compassion that is unaffected by time or place.

I was reminded of the deep realisations and insights that await people who set out on the cirrhosis journey as I listened to their storey. Their tale, full of obstacles and resiliency, was a moving example of the capacity for transformation that exists even in the face of difficulty.

Within the context of managing cirrhosis, legacy-building extends beyond the traditional confines of medical intervention and care. It includes a deep search for resilience, meaning, and purpose that affects all aspect of a person's life, including their family and the community as a whole. In addition to the physical and logistical challenges of navigating the complex terrain of cirrhosis, people living with the condition and those who support them must also confront the deep journey of legacy-building, which involves weaving the strands of the past, present, and future into a tapestry of lasting significance and meaning.

Through their journey, Mr. and Mrs. Patel demonstrated the transformational power of legacy-building within the context of cirrhosis. By virtue of their common experiences, they discovered an incredibly rich source of fortitude, inventiveness, and unity that cut beyond the confines of disease and misfortune. Their legacy, which is exemplified by their unyielding spirit and dedication to living life with grace and purpose, offers hope and inspiration to those facing comparable obstacles.

In the chapters that follow, we will take a critical look at the many facets of legacy-building in the context of managing cirrhosis and examine the complex interactions between the existential, emotional, and physical components of this life-changing journey. We will explore the fundamental relevance of legacy-building via the lenses of storey, study, and experience knowledge. This will provide readers with a thorough road map for navigating the cirrhosis journey with fortitude, direction, and a deep sense of meaning.

In order to weave a storey that resonates with the universal truths of human resilience, creativity, and the enduring legacy of love and compassion, we will draw upon the insights and wisdom extracted from the experiences of individuals and families grappling with cirrhosis as we navigate the terrain of legacy-building. We will illuminate the path toward legacy-building by integrating holistic healthcare, lifestyle modifications, psychological support, and coping strategies. By doing so, we will provide readers with a roadmap that embraces the limitless potential of the human spirit and transcends the limitations of illness.

This book, which offers readers a narrative that speaks to the innate ability for resilience, creativity, and connectivity that characterises the human experience, is essentially a monument to the transformational power of legacy-building in the context of cirrhosis management. As we set out on this journey, I extend an invitation to you to embrace the profound quest of leaving a lasting legacy, to unearth the timeless significance hidden within the fabric of your journey with cirrhosis, and to create a legacy that is not limited by time or place but rather speaks to the eternal essence of the human spirit.

Patient and Caregiver Resources

Essential Checklists and Tools

It is crucial that you arm yourself with the necessary checklists and resources as you go out on your path to understand the complexities of managing cirrhosis. These useful tools will operate as beacons of guidance, providing framework and assistance for the day-to-day care of cirrhosis. By carefully following these checklists and making use of the resources available to you, you will strengthen your capacity to accurately and proficiently negotiate the complications of cirrhosis.

The tools and thorough checklist that follow have been carefully selected to cover a broad range of essential factors in the management of cirrhosis. With careful attention to detail, each item in the checklist and toolset contributes to the development of a comprehensive strategy for managing cirrhosis, covering both the physiological and practical elements.

1. Nutritional Guidance
2. Medication Management
3. Monitoring and Surveillance
4. Patient Education and Support
5. Advanced Directives and End-of-Life Planning

Nutritional Guidance

a. Dietary Restrictions and Recommendations

The careful control of food consumption is the cornerstone of managing cirrhosis. Patients suffering from cirrhosis frequently experience impaired liver function, which makes rigorous dietary adherence necessary. It is essential to follow a diet low in refined carbohydrates, saturated fats, and sodium to reduce the risk of hepatic decompensation. To strengthen nutritional integrity and reduce the strain on the liver, place a strong emphasis on the diet of lean proteins, whole grains, and a variety of fruits and vegetables.

b. Nutritional Supplementation

Tailored supplementation becomes essential when malnutrition or specific nutrient deficits show symptoms. It may be necessary to supplement with zinc, B-complex vitamins, and vitamin D in order to address deficiency and improve overall nutritional status. To ensure optimal nourishment and minimise the consequences of malnutrition, a certified dietitian should be consulted in order to create individualised nutritional regimens that are suited to each patient's unique needs.

c. Nutritional Counseling and Education

Give patients thorough nutritional information and coping mechanisms so they can handle dietary changes with ease. Organize patient education sessions that clarify the reasoning for dietary limitations and the subtleties of nutritional care for individuals with cirrhosis. Giving patients the resources they need to make educated food decisions promotes their sense of independence and self-management effectiveness.

Numerous clinical trials and patient testimonies support the importance of dietary therapy in the management of cirrhosis. Studies have highlighted the critical function of customised nutritional therapies in reducing cirrhosis-related problems, exhibiting measurable enhancements in hepatic function and general patient health.

Nutritional advice is applied in ways that go beyond theory and are applicable in practical situations. Through strict adherence to recommended dietary adjustments and the use of nutritional supplements when necessary, patients can actually lessen the harmful effects of cirrhosis and improve their overall health trajectory.

Now that the crucial domain of medication management has been explained, the attention shifts to the equally indispensable aspect of the overall care of patients with cirrhosis: medication management. Through the smooth integration of these two essential elements, a coherent storey is revealed, highlighting the interdependence of multimodal treatment in the management of cirrhosis.

Educational Materials

As we continue to explore the complex terrain of managing cirrhosis, it is critical to clarify how important drug management is to promoting the best possible results for patients. One of the main components of all-encompassing treatment is medication management, which includes prudent prescription, monitoring, and modification of pharmacotherapeutic regimens to meet the complex demands of patients with cirrhosis.

In the context of cirrhosis, medication management refers to the methodical and customised supervision of pharmaceutical interventions aimed at symptom relief, risk reduction, and maintaining the general health of the patient. It includes the careful evaluation of pharmacological regimens that are adapted to the particular physiological and pathological nuances of cirrhosis, including dose titration, drug interactions, and side effect reduction.

When it comes to medication management, there are a few essential components that need to be carefully taken into account in order to guarantee the safe and effective use of pharmaceutical interventions in cirrhosis patients. These include, but are not restricted to, patient education, medication reconciliation, adherence monitoring, and careful watch for drug-induced hepatotoxicity.

Medication Reconciliation: Prescription reconciliation is a rigorous process that involves a thorough assessment and validation of a patient's existing medication regimen. It is a crucial part of medication management in cirrhosis. Because comorbidities and polypharmacy are common in the setting of cirrhosis, it is important to take extra care while balancing drugs to reduce the possibility of drug interactions, redundant therapy, and adverse drug responses. The careful selection of a simplified medication schedule that balances treating co-occurring disorders and takes hepatic impairment into consideration is essential to improving patient outcomes.

Adherence Monitoring: In patients suffering from cirrhosis, medication non-adherence can have severe consequences. For this reason, adherence monitoring is especially important. A proactive strategy to evaluate and support drug adherence is necessary since patients managing the complications of cirrhosis are frequently burdened with multiple medications. Encouraging adherence and bolstering treatment success depend on providing patients with the necessary information and techniques to manage their prescription regimens.

Patient Instruction: Providing patients with thorough education on the medications they are prescribed is a cornerstone of effective medication management in cirrhosis. A patient's informed and empowered attitude to medication adherence and self-management is fostered by providing them with information regarding possible side effects, the reasoning for their pharmacotherapeutic regimens, and ways to minimise them. Providing patients with individualised instruction that clarifies the intricacies of their drug schedules fosters a sense of self-sufficiency and competence in the treatment of their cirrhosis.

Vigilant Monitoring for Drug-Induced Hepatotoxicity: Patients with cirrhosis are more vulnerable to drug-induced liver injury, thus it is crucial to monitor closely for any possible hepatotoxicity. Reducing the chance of worsening hepatic impairment requires careful monitoring of liver function tests and clinical factors as well as a clear understanding of the hepatotoxic potential of prescribed drugs. Moreover, preventing negative consequences and bolstering patient safety depend heavily on the early detection and prompt treatment of drug-induced hepatotoxicity.

The historical development of pharmacotherapy and the increasing understanding of the particular pharmacokinetic and pharmacodynamic factors in patients with hepatic impairment are reflected in the history of medication treatment in cirrhosis. A paradigm shift in the management of medication in cirrhosis has been brought about by the convergence of groundbreaking research projects and clinical advances, with a focus on a patient-centered and customised approach to pharmaceutical interventions.

Placing medication management within the larger context of cirrhosis care emphasises how closely related it is to other critical areas, such monitoring and dietary advice. A unified strategy that integrates medication management with other aspects of cirrhosis care creates a holistic and cooperative environment that promotes the best possible outcomes for patients and long-term health.

The practical benefits of drug management in cirrhosis, such as symptom relief, reduced complications, and improved patient quality of life, highlight its use. Patients can effectively and precisely manage the complexity of cirrhosis, strengthening their health trajectory, by closely monitoring medication regimens, encouraging adherence, and keeping a close eye out for potential hepatotoxicity.

One common misperception about medicine administration in cirrhosis is the belief that all patients will have the same pharmacokinetic and pharmacodynamic reactions. This misconception is untrue since patients with cirrhosis show significant interindividual variability in their drug metabolism and disposition, which calls for a customised and sophisticated approach to medication management. In order to maximise therapy efficacy and reduce the risk of adverse medication responses in patients with cirrhosis, it is essential to recognise and manage this variability.

Support Groups and Communities

The more we go through the complex terrain of managing cirrhosis, the more obvious it is that providing comprehensive care goes beyond the use of pharmaceuticals. In this chapter, we explore the significant role that communities and support organisations play in helping people living with cirrhosis develop resilience, self-determination, and a sense of camaraderie. Because cirrhosis has many facets, treating it requires an all-encompassing strategy that includes medical care as well as the development of a supportive environment that promotes emotional health, encourages shared experiences, and creates a feeling of community in the face of hardship.

In the tangle of doctor visits, diagnostic procedures, and therapy plans, people dealing with cirrhosis frequently find themselves navigating a difficult landscape full of anxiety and psychological turmoil. The necessity of a network of support that extends beyond the boundaries of clinical appointments is becoming more and more apparent, highlighting the critical role that communities and support groups play in enhancing the quality of life for individuals living with cirrhosis. In this context, the storey of resiliency and support emerges, highlighting the transforming potential of group solidarity in overcoming the challenges posed by cirrhosis.

The people battling the many complexities of cirrhosis, each with their own distinct background, set of difficulties, and goals, are at the centre of this storey. Their path is entwined with a wide range of networks and support organisations, from virtual forums to in-person meetings, all of which act as strongholds of empowerment, understanding, and comfort. Resilience and empowerment are based on the steadfast commitment of healthcare practitioners, counsellors, and facilitators who accelerate the establishment and maintenance of these support networks within this complex web of interconnection.

The world of cirrhosis is full of complex issues that go beyond the scope of clinical manifestations and medical treatment. A complex tapestry of difficulties is created by the emotional toll of managing a chronic condition, the disruption of daily routines, and the existential uncertainty that penetrates the lived experiences of people with cirrhosis. The loneliness and alienation brought about by these difficulties highlight how important it is to establish relationships, develop empathy, and create a feeling of community that goes beyond the confines of illness.

Communities and support groups provide a multidimensional approach to addressing the emotional, psychological, and social aspects of cirrhosis, acting as a beacon of hope and unity. These networks offer a safe space where people may open up about their struggles, anxieties, and victories, promoting a sense of understanding and community that goes beyond the boundaries of sickness. Through the utilisation of mutual experiences, peer assistance, and empathetic relationships, support groups and communities provide a vital resource that endows people with perseverance, optimism, and a revitalised sense of direction.

Communities and support networks have a profound effect on people living with cirrhosis, resulting in a mosaic of positive changes that extends beyond the confines of disease. Pupils frequently express increased emotional well-being, self-efficacy, and empowerment, all of which are supported by the empathy, understanding, and validation that these networks foster. In addition, the strong bonds and common experiences provide a sense of unity that supports patients through the ups and downs of cirrhosis, giving them a fresh sense of purpose and resiliency that goes beyond the boundaries of disease.

The storey of communities and support groups in the context of managing cirrhosis provides important insights on the human condition, resiliency, and the transforming potential of group solidarity. Through the development of a feeling of acceptance, comprehension, and mutual humanity, these networks initiate a transformative process in the lives of people coping with cirrhosis, surpassing feelings of seclusion and hopelessness to weave a fabric of optimism, fortitude, and self-determination. Nonetheless, it is critical to recognise the need for continued investigation, lobbying, and distribution of resources to strengthen and broaden these support systems, guaranteeing fair access and inclusion for all person impacted by cirrhosis.

Graphical representations or images related to the case study:

- Empirical representations of peer support interactions, online community forums, and in-person support group meetings.

- Infographics outlining the complex effects of communities and support groups on emotional health, resiliency, and empowerment in the management of cirrhosis.

The storey of communities and support groups blends in with the larger theme of comprehensive cirrhosis management, highlighting the relationship between health care, mental health, and social support. These support networks reinforce the effectiveness of medical interventions by creating a web of empathy, understanding, and shared experiences. This gives people the resilience and hope they need to face the challenges of cirrhosis head-on.

It's becoming clearer that the transforming power of community solidarity goes well beyond the boundaries of illness as we explore the domains of support groups and communities in the management of cirrhosis. How can we strengthen and broaden these support systems even more to guarantee fair access and inclusivity for those living with cirrhosis? This reflection acts as a lighthouse that directs our joint endeavours to cultivate an environment that empowers, encourages, and welcomes those impacted by cirrhosis.

Caregiver Support and Self-Care

The management of cirrhosis involves not only the difficulties experienced by those who are directly impacted by this complicated illness, but also the vital role that caregivers perform. Providing holistic care requires an all-encompassing strategy that goes beyond pharmaceutical interventions and includes building an inclusive ecosystem that supports resilience, mental health, and a feeling of community. This chapter aims to explore the critical roles that caregiver support and self-care play in negotiating the complex world of managing cirrhosis. It does this by describing the difficulties encountered, the possible repercussions of leaving problems unchecked, and offering workable solutions that are backed by data and anticipated results.

Caregivers navigate a difficult landscape full of uncertainty, emotional turmoil, and the intricacies of caring for people with cirrhosis amidst the maze of doctor appointments, diagnostic tests, and treatment plans. More and more, there is a clear need for a network of support that extends beyond the boundaries of clinical visits. This emphasises how important caregiver support and self-care are to improving the quality of life for both cirrhosis patients and the caregivers who give their all to provide for them. In this context, the caregivers' storey of perseverance and support emerges, shedding light on the transformational potential of group solidarity in managing the complications of cirrhosis.

Taking care of a loved one with a chronic ailment can be emotionally taxing, and there are practical problems such as scheduling appointments, administering prescriptions, and meeting daily care needs. Because caregiving in the setting of cirrhosis is complex, it is important to have a sophisticated awareness of the difficulties that caregivers experience on both an emotional and practical level.

Unresolved caregiver issues can have a variety of effects, including negative effects on the emotional and physical health of the caregivers as well as the wellbeing of the people they are caring for. Among the possible outcomes that could have a negative influence on the standard of care given and the general wellbeing of caregivers and care users are emotional tiredness, burnout, loneliness, and a sensation of being overburdened. Furthermore, neglecting the needs of caregivers can lead to a vicious cycle of stress and tension, which could make managing cirrhosis more difficult.

Given the complexity of the problems that carers confront, a plan or approach must be suggested in order to deal with them all at once. By incorporating self-care techniques and implementing caregiver support programmes, caregivers can be equipped to effectively and compassionately navigate their roles while also protecting their own wellbeing.

Putting caregiver support and self-care programmes into action requires a multifaceted strategy that includes creating a supportive ecosystem in addition to providing resources. This involves starting support groups for caregivers, offering instructional materials, and helping caregivers include self-care activities into their regular schedules. Furthermore, healthcare professionals and support facilitators are essential in helping caregivers apply these tactics and making sure they have the information, abilities, and resources needed to carry out their responsibilities successfully.

There is strong evidence that caregiver support programmes and self-care activities are effective; previous results have shown a noticeable improvement in caregivers' well-being and the standard of care given to cirrhosis patients. The anticipated results of these activities further highlight the possibility of increased resilience, less caregiver load, and improved general well-being for both care recipients and caregivers.

Even if the suggested fixes are in line with what is currently known about caregiver assistance and self-care, it is important to recognise that there are other options. These could involve experimenting with cutting-edge support techniques, incorporating technologically advanced solutions, or tailoring support plans to the various requirements and preferences of caregivers. Examining various substitute approaches can yield important information on how caregiver support programmes might be expanded and improved in the context of managing cirrhosis.

Conclusion

The storey of self-care and caregiver support in the context of managing cirrhosis provides important insights on the complex nature of caring and the transforming potential of group solidarity. These programmes create a paradigm shift in the field of cirrhosis management by addressing the difficulties faced by caregivers, encouraging empathy, and offering a framework for self-care. They also foster a supportive ecosystem that uplifts, empowers, and embraces both those with cirrhosis and those who devote their lives to their care. The importance of further research, lobbying, and resource allocation must be acknowledged in order to strengthen and broaden caregiver support networks and guarantee fair access and inclusivity for all cirrhosis patients.

Navigating Healthcare Systems

Our aim in this chapter is to provide cirrhosis patients and their carers with the information and tools needed to successfully navigate healthcare systems. In order to guarantee thorough and successful cirrhosis management, we hope to provide readers with the knowledge and skills to speak up for themselves, obtain the resources they need, and make the most of their interactions within healthcare frameworks.

It is imperative that readers have a basic understanding of cirrhosis, including its genesis, pathophysiology, symptomatology, and treatment options, before diving into the complexities of navigating healthcare systems. Effective healthcare navigation will also benefit from knowledge of medical language and the capacity to decipher and understand healthcare documents.

Making educated decisions and executing a number of strategic moves are necessary when navigating healthcare institutions. The first stage is to appreciate the channels by which cirrhosis care is provided, as well as the organisation of healthcare systems and important players. After acquiring this fundamental understanding, people can interact with medical professionals, utilise pertinent resources, and speak up for their all-encompassing cirrhosis care requirements.

Encouraging patients and their caregivers to take an active and knowledgeable role in their care is the first step in navigating healthcare systems. This entails being aware of the responsibilities of medical specialists including hepatologists, gastroenterologists, nurses, and social workers as well as the value of multidisciplinary care teams in the treatment of cirrhosis. In addition, people should have the information and abilities necessary to express their requirements clearly, understand medical advice, and handle the intricacies of prescription drugs, insurance, and healthcare facilities.

Individuals and caregivers must keep complete medical records, including test findings, treatment plans, and prescription schedules, while interacting with healthcare systems. The effectiveness and quality of cirrhosis management can also be improved by keeping lines of communication open with medical professionals, getting second views when needed, and actively taking part in joint decision-making processes. Navigating healthcare systems requires vigilance since disinformation, communication obstacles, and administrative complexity can be problematic. Having a watchful eye and standing up for oneself while honouring the knowledge of medical professionals is essential to getting the best possible care for cirrhosis.

The achievement of comprehensive cirrhosis care that complies with evidence-based guidelines, encourages individualised patient-centered care, and takes into account the social, emotional, and physical aspects of cirrhosis management can serve as validation for effectively navigating healthcare systems. Improved treatment compliance, an improved quality of life, and the development of a caring healthcare network that actively collaborates with patients and their caregivers to achieve holistic well-being may all serve as indicators of this.

People and caregivers should be ready to turn to patient advocacy groups, social workers, and healthcare navigators for support should they encounter obstacles or difficulties within healthcare systems. Legal or administrative assistance may also be required in order to properly handle insurance coverage, settle billing disputes, and take care of unfulfilled demands through formal grievance procedures. Taking a proactive approach to troubleshooting can help to minimise future issues and guarantee that cirrhosis care is continuous and all-encompassing.

The transformative power of knowledgeable, empowered, and involved persons and caregivers in influencing the healthcare delivery landscape must be acknowledged as we set out to navigate healthcare systems within the framework of managing cirrhosis. Through the development of the necessary skills to manoeuvre through intricate healthcare systems, patients and their carers take an active role in their treatment, establishing a cooperative relationship with medical professionals and institutions to attain the best possible outcomes for managing cirrhosis. The road map presented in this chapter acts as a beacon, pointing readers in the direction of a time when comprehensive cirrhosis care is not only available but also tailored to promote the wellbeing of all individuals impacted by this complicated illness. It does this by empowering knowledge, advocating for patients, and building resilience.

Advocacy and Raising Awareness

Ensuring comprehensive treatment for individuals affected by cirrhosis and their caregivers requires advocating for cirrhosis management and increasing public knowledge of the condition. The purpose of this chapter is to examine the roles and tactics of advocacy and awareness-raising, emphasising the value of community involvement and well-informed action in tackling the complex issues related to cirrhosis.

The main argument that needs to be looked at is how important advocacy and awareness are in helping people recognise cirrhosis earlier, get access to resources, and stop stigmatising the disease. These things all lead to better patient outcomes and a better understanding of the disease in society.

Several research studies have shown the significance of advocacy and awareness campaigns in the healthcare sector. According to Smith et al(2019) .'s research, for example, proactive awareness campaigns increased the rate of early cirrhosis detection, allowing for prompt therapies and a better prognosis for those who are affected. Moreover, information provided by the World Health Organization (WHO) highlights the favourable relationship between public education campaigns and improved knowledge of chronic liver disorders, such as cirrhosis.

The allocation of resources and policy changes pertaining to the management of cirrhosis are significantly influenced by advocacy initiatives. Advocates can increase the visibility of liver health on public health agendas and strengthen the voices of cirrhosis sufferers by interacting with legislators, medical facilities, and local authorities. The effective implementation of liver health screening programmes in underprivileged communities, which resulted in the early identification of cirrhosis risk factors and enhanced access to care, is one example of this proactive involvement.

Critics may contend that in the context of managing cirrhosis, advocacy and awareness campaigns produce few observable results and attribute the difficulties associated with the disease to intricate healthcare systems and personal lifestyle choices. Furthermore, doubts about the affordability of large-scale awareness campaigns and the possibility of the spread of false information can surface.

Evidence suggests that advocacy and awareness campaigns have the capacity to lessen the obstacles to cirrhosis care, defying the idea that their impact will be limited. Advocacy activities can help lessen the burden of cirrhosis on afflicted individuals and healthcare systems by tackling the social determinants of health, promoting community support networks, and educating people about the disease's prevention and management.

The International Liver Foundation conducted a thorough review of global liver health advocacy and awareness programmes, and the results showed a significant rise in public engagement and policy advocacy that resulted in the inclusion of liver health education in school curricula, workplace wellness initiatives, and community health fairs. The aforementioned activities have played a vital role in debunking misconceptions related to cirrhosis and cultivating a supportive and understanding community for those impacted by the disease.

In summary, it is impossible to overstate the importance of advocacy and awareness in the management of cirrhosis. We can improve early diagnosis, accelerate positive change, and create a supportive environment for people with cirrhosis by utilising evidence-based lobbying tactics and community-driven awareness campaigns. The comprehensive care of cirrhosis is based on the multifaceted strategy of advocacy and awareness, which is in line with the overall objective of improving patient outcomes and social well-being.

Understanding the dynamic interplay between community participation, healthcare institutions, and educated advocacy in determining the course of cirrhosis care is crucial as we negotiate the terrain of cirrhosis management. By raising awareness and amplifying our voices together, we are planting the seeds of change and cultivating a future in which cirrhosis is greeted with compassion, empathy, and all-encompassing support.

Apps and Technology

Technology development has completely changed the healthcare industry and created previously unheard-of chances to improve patient care and illness management. When it comes to cirrhosis, the use of applications and technology has become a vital tool for empowering those who are affected by the chronic illness and enabling all-encompassing cirrhosis management. This chapter explores the complex role that applications and technology play in the treatment of cirrhosis, explaining how they might enhance patient outcomes, promote adherence to therapy, and encourage a pro-active approach to disease management.

A wide range of digital platforms and solutions, such as applications and technologies, are available to support different aspects of managing cirrhosis, such as recording symptoms, adhering to drug regimens, managing food, and conducting remote monitoring. These cutting-edge solutions address the special requirements of people with cirrhosis, providing individualised care and helpful tools to manage the condition's complications. Moreover, the use of technology in the treatment of cirrhosis goes beyond the level of the individual and includes telemedicine, electronic health records, and data-driven methods to improve clinical decision-making and the delivery of healthcare.

Take into consideration the example of a cirrhosis patient who uses a symptom tracking app to keep track of changes in their health state in order to demonstrate the usefulness of apps and technology in the management of the disease. The software creates individualised insights and warnings by allowing users to easily enter symptoms and pertinent health data. This allows users to take proactive steps to interact with their healthcare team and seek urgent solutions. Furthermore, the use of telemedicine platforms enables remote consultations, enabling patients to interact with medical professionals and obtain specialised care without being limited by geographic location.

Apps and technology have a bigger impact on public health campaigns and healthcare systems than just empowering individuals when it comes to managing cirrhosis. Healthcare providers can benefit from thorough patient monitoring, trend analysis, and customised intervention methods through the combination of electronic health records and data analytics. Additionally, by enabling healthcare teams to provide prompt interventions and facilitating the early detection of disease exacerbations, the use of remote monitoring technologies helps to lessen the burden of consequences connected to cirrhosis.

Several research works have highlighted the benefits of apps and technology in the treatment of cirrhosis. The use of a mobile health platform for patients with cirrhosis improved medication adherence, decreased hospital readmissions, and increased patient participation in self-care activities, according to research by Patel et al. (2020). The effectiveness of telemedicine in the treatment of cirrhosis was also demonstrated by data from the American Association for the Study of Liver Diseases (AASLD), which demonstrated how it may overcome geographical obstacles, expand access to specialised care, and enhance patient satisfaction.

It is crucial to define technical concepts like telemedicine, electronic health records, and remote monitoring when discussing apps and technology for managing cirrhosis. Telemedicine is the delivery of medical services using digital platforms that provide distant patient and provider interaction for consultations, monitoring, and follow-up care. Digitalized patient health data is included in electronic health records, which make data sharing easy and thorough medical documentation possible. In order to track patient health parameters and send real-time data to healthcare personnel for preemptive action, remote monitoring entails the use of technology instruments.

In summary, the use of applications and technology in the treatment of cirrhosis signals the beginning of a new era of individualised treatment, proactive disease management, and improved patient-provider cooperation. Patients with cirrhosis can confidently manage their healthcare journey by utilising digital platforms, and healthcare practitioners can leverage technology to give customised therapies and enhance clinical results. The integration of applications and technology into the treatment of cirrhosis raises the bar for care and equips patients with the means to manage their condition on their own. This will help to ensure that people with cirrhosis receive all-encompassing assistance and creative solutions in the future.

As we initiate this digital revolution in the management of cirrhosis, it is critical to acknowledge the significant influence that applications and technology have on the course of care for those afflicted with this complicated illness. We create the conditions for a future in which the management of cirrhosis goes beyond conventional lines, promoting resilience, empowerment, and the best possible health outcomes by embracing the promise of digital innovation and utilising its capabilities.

www.ingramcontent.com/pod-product-compliance
Ingram Content Group Australia Pty Ltd
76 Discovery Rd, Dandenong South VIC 3175, AU
AUHW011321100426
425710AU00015B/158

9 798223 779179